Nephew
John John (Jo)
stay focus
keep your eyes on
sing a song
Eyes are watching you!
I love you very much
Johnathan.

Love
Always.
E.

It's All about

Me!

Becoming a Conscious Eater

by
Edna Ellen Elizabeth Harris-Davis

authorHOUSE®

AuthorHouse™
1663 Liberty Drive, Suite 200
Bloomington, IN 47403
www.authorhouse.com
Phone: 1-800-839-8640

First published by AuthorHouse 3/11/2010

ISBN: 978-1-4490-0835-2 (sc)

Library of Congress Control Number: 2010901396

Printed in the United States of America
Bloomington, Indiana

This book is printed on acid-free paper.

Illustrations #1, 2, 3 by Rose Lester
Illustration # 4 by ©Getty Images/Dynamic Group
Illustration #5 by ©Getty Images/Jupiter Images
Diagrams by Edna Davis
Cover Design by Janelle Gonyea
Front Cover Picture by ©iStockphoto.com/hidesy
Back Cover Picture by ©iStockphoto.com/digitalskillet

Disclaimer

Information contained in this book should not be used as a substitute for professional recommendation or advice nor used as a weight-loss program. Readers must consult their health care provider including private physician on chronic symptoms, illnesses, or diseases, including prevention and treatment programs. If further services are needed, readers should seek a competent professional to address their weight and/or chronic disease management needs and concerns. The author or other individuals involved with developing this book shall not be liable or responsible for any loss, injury, or damage allegedly arising from any information or suggestions in this book.

It's All about Me! is not endorsed or supported by any religious organization, institution, association, support groups, or any other groups not mentioned here.

1. Conscious Eating 2. Unconscious Eating 3. Spiritual Food 4. Mind and Body 5. Overeating 6. Overweight 7. Purpose in Life 8. Poetry 9. Eat to Live

IT'S ALL ABOUT ME!
BECOMING A CONSCIOUS EATER

CONTENTS

Part 1: Awareness
Ground Zero

Part 2: Knowledge
Plant the Seeds

Part 3: Skills
Grow a Garden

DEDICATIONS

I dedicate this book to my pen pal, Sister Sherra, of 26 years. Over the years, I believe we were in competition over who wrote the longest letters. Well, consider this book as my letter to you, and so far I am winning.

I dedicate this book to my husband who has been the head of our family by leading and supporting me and our sons over the years.

I dedicate this book to my two sons. When you are older and able to understand this book, I hope it encourages you to make conscious decisions in all your endeavors, including eating.

The poem I dedicate to my nephew Chris—the first Harris grandchild. Turn this thing around.

I dedicate my love to all the Harris grandchildren. You are our prosperity for generations to come. Our collective eyes are watching you.

I dedicate this book to all my ancestors who came before me and worked diligently in very challenging eras. Many of them endured and overcame the struggles of life and dreamed of successes that are alive in me today.

I dedicate this book to all those who struggle with overeating, overweight, unconscious eating, and unhealthy living – living without a purpose. I know your struggles. Some readers may be looking for ways to be a conscious eater with physical and/or spiritual food. I hope and pray you will find what you are looking for.

I dedicate this book to the young and the old, but especially the young people that have slipped away too soon in this lifetime because they did not experience the self awareness, knowledge and skills of conscious eating both physically and spiritually.

THANK YOU!

- ❖ I want to thank my awesome GOD! Thy kingdom come. Thy will be done *on earth* as it is in heaven.
- ❖ I want to thank my Cousin who shared his God-given wisdom with me and helped me to open my eyes. Boy, was I sleeping.
- ❖ I want to thank my Parents, who said, "Go to school and get a degree and then do what you want to do." I have earned several degrees over the years, and those experiences prepared me. Now I know my purpose in life. I am so glad I did not let another year go by—by sleeping! However, after reading this book, I hope my parents will have a spiritual understanding of why I always said, **"I don't want to grow up!"**
- ❖ I want to thank my Two Church Families, who have given me a solid foundation in God's Word. Through church experiences and relationships, I was able to survive some difficult years. God's words are truer to me now than ever before.
- ❖ I want to thank my Sister for her love and support throughout the years, including being the family doctor and asking the right questions.
- ❖ I want to thank my Older Brother for the many discussions we continue to have about "Just push away from the table!" and "Just say NO!"
- ❖ I want to thank my Younger Brother for all his love, and I hope one day he will *wake up* and see all the many talents God has given him. Remember, it's all about me! Turn it around.
- ❖ I want to thank my Special Friends, who helped me in my journey of becoming a conscious eater.
- ❖ I want to thank all who provided valuable feedback in the making of this book.
- ❖ I want to thank my professor, who turned the pages with me in obtaining a worldview of diet, nutrition and counseling. We kept an open mind and I hope so many health professionals will do the same.

PREFACE

"The just shall live by faith."
Romans 1:17

A just man does not need laws. The Lord will create in you a new heart, a new mind and a new spirit. Therefore, the laws are written in your heart and you do them naturally. (Read the book *Overcoming Yourself: A journey toward self improvement and oneness* to get a better understanding of *It's All about Me: Becoming a Conscious Eater*.)

"Faith is the substance of things hoped for
and the evidence of things not seen."
Hebrews 12:1

If being healthy is your hope and being a healthy individual is the outcome then believe it and receive it. Walk by faith and not by sight. Walking by faith is not a physical action, it is a spiritual one. Build your mind up (the conscious mind—the unseen thing) to be the leader of this great body or gift God created for you. "Walk in the SPIRIT (the unseen thing) and ye shall not fulfill the lust of the flesh." Galatians 5:16

Throughout this book, the **CONSCIOUS MIND** and the **UNCONSCIOUS MIND** will be used interchangeably with **PARENT** and **CHILD** and **MIND** and **BODY**, respectively. These words are used to help the reader to understand the dynamics of conscious and unconscious eating. The descriptive examples and illustrations throughout the book will help the reader to understand the main concepts of this book.

"Wisdom is the principal thing: therefore get wisdom:
and with all thy getting, get an understanding."
Proverb 4:7

After reading this book, I hope you experience a change; your change may come sooner or later. Whatever your path, I urge you to be a hearer and put the book down and *DO* something to become a *CONSCIOUS EATER*. After all, it's all about You!

ABOUT THIS BOOK

While a diet plan and/or nutrition therapy is good, this book is not about either. *It's All about Me!* is about your relationship with God—a Higher Power—and becoming a conscious eater.

In this book, you will read about my struggles with food. In my struggles, I knew something was wrong or went wrong, but I did not know how to fix it. My breakthrough occurred when I read *Overcoming Yourself: A journey toward self improvement and oneness*. I began to see clearly the consciousness and unconsciousness concepts, and I understood my life struggles immediately, including eating unconsciously.

Over the years as a dietitian, I struggled as a professional to truly help people prevent chronic diseases, i.e., heart disease, cancer, diabetes, and obesity. I saw the dietetic profession work diligently in research and practice. Also, I saw the sincerity of the professionals who gave the information and those who received it. Yet, oftentimes there was a disconnect. A disconnect with both the messenger and the receiver and also with the receiver and putting the messages into action.

Like I said before, the diet plans, the nutrition therapy, and the research behind them may be good. However, if the person's **state of mind** is not ready and prepared to receive it, then it is worthless. So, how does a person have the right state of mind to receive these good messages and put them into action? Overcome yourself! When a person has a better understanding of consciousness and unconsciousness, then I believe most people can hear those good messages and apply them to their life and lifestyle.

Conscious eating is a physical awareness of bodily functions and the environment during the eating process so that one knows when to stop the process because the body has achieved a level of being comfortably full and obtained enough energy to carry out daily activities to fulfill one's purpose in life.

Conscious eating is a spiritual awareness of God's word as a source of spiritual food. It includes a desire to meditate on God's word that will feed, build and restore a person's mind and body in order to fulfill one's purpose in life.

My prayer and hope is that the reader increases his or her physical and spiritual awareness through the Ground Zero Process by developing a parent-child relationship with oneself when consuming food. Through this awareness, I hope you can expand your knowledge of conscious eating through planting new seeds and images in your mind. As a result of your awareness and knowledge, I hope you will apply the skills needed to become a conscious eater. Enjoy!

IT'S ALL ABOUT ME!

MY STRUGGLE

When I was a child, I can remember episodes of overeating. Some earlier episodes occurred on Fridays and Saturdays when my mom made her famous chocolate chip cookies. My siblings and I would eat cookies when they first came out of the oven. They melted in my mouth, leaving a pleasurable experience for all my senses: eyes seeing the melted chocolate with every bite; nose smelling the aroma of fresh-baked cookies; fingers feeling the warmth and softness of the cookie—like a nice warm pillow; tongue and taste buds full of saliva waiting for the sweetness of every bite; and the ears that heard the joyful conversation of others who were experiencing the same.

Seeing the cookies on the counter was temptation to eat more cookies. Although the experience was not the same as the cookies coming out of the oven, the cookies were *there*. They were *there* on the counter, cooling off. The smell was still lingering in the air. The experience is still fresh in my mind. The temptation of wanting more cookies was more than a child could handle, both physically and spiritually. Physically, eating too many cookies was too much for this child's small body. Spiritually, as a child, I was a lamb drawn by the temptation of eating more cookies, not knowing the dangers behind the temptation. The cookies were still *there* in the house over the weekend, in that special container. My hands were not my own. My fingers were not my own. I see myself unconsciously grabbing a couple of cookies trying to make as little noise as possible in the middle of the night, and not asking for an adult's permission. I would sneak the cookies away, but all true consciousness of knowing right from wrong was not there. What was *there* was temptation. What was *there* was the lure of pleasure. What was *there* was cruise control—autopilot. What was *there* was the cookie that gave me the illusion of becoming my friend. What was *there* was the beginning of my unconscious state of mind. Eating a few cookies at a family gathering monitored by adults turned into eating several cookies unnoticed without supervision, to include several times during the day and night in hiding places.

Unconscious eating became my struggle over the next thirty years. Unconscious eating gave me an illusion that everything was going to be all right—a false pleasure and a way to deal with the pain or struggles of life. I ate to stay up in the middle of the night and study for exams. I ate to get over a breakup with a boyfriend. I ate to laugh and have fun with my girlfriends/sisters. I ate and drank in the car as I ran errands. I ate when I finished major projects, to celebrate my accomplishments. I ate when there were free samples in the grocery store or the food court in the mall. I ate when my boyfriend cooked for me, and consumed large portions of food to show my appreciation. I ate to grieve. I ate to be happy and avoid being lonely. Food became my friend. This was my pleasure over the years. It was *there*. Food was *there*. It was there and sometimes there too much, which caused me to overeat, eating more calories than my body truly needed or would burn off. Food eventually became my drug of choice to deal with the struggles of life, i.e., frustrations of the job, loneliness, financial woes, marital and family challenges, car troubles, and even happiness.

Now looking back, I perceived that I was lonely and in pain. This false perception was a link to the desire of having more of this food - Having more of this drug. Having more of this foggy brain that gives you a state of mind not to think or feel pain, loneliness, or struggles of life. Or even true happiness when it comes. In this stupor, the body wants to be on cruise control—on autopilot—going through the motions in an inertia-like existence—accepting the mundane experiences of life. I was unconscious not only in eating but in every aspect of my life. My life became mundane, and I expected and wanted that life until I became conscious of that existence. Now I am conscious and aware of my eating habits and purpose in life. Best of all, I realize that God is with me, and He was **there** all the time, waiting to remove the scales from my eyes and for me to accept His love.

PART 1:
AWARENESS
GROUND ZERO

CHAPTER 1
Acknowledgments

Before you can overcome and be a conscious eater,
you must first acknowledge there is a problem!

So many times, we have found ourselves struggling with our eating habits. We eat late at night; we eat when we are stressed; we eat when we are worried; we eat when we are happy; we eat when we are bored; we eat because someone said, "It's time to eat," or "Try this, it tastes so good!" We eat to stay up longer; we eat because it is a routine; we eat because someone else is eating; we overeat; we eat because there is a party; we eat snacks because there is nothing prepared to eat. We eat standing up or walking; we eat while on the telephone; we eat while watching television; we eat because we think the food is going to spoil or it will become too soggy; we eat out of competition; we eat at the computer; we eat after an accomplishment. We eat when we are rushed; we eat while cooking; we eat while standing in front of the refrigerator or the kitchen cabinets; we eat just because, just because, just because. Then we wonder why so many of us have chronic illnesses. Many of these diseases are preventable. Before we can prevent chronic diseases or poor eating habits, we must first realize that there is a problem. If you see yourself "eating just because …" then you may be an unconscious eater. If so, acknowledge your unconscious eating habits and *do* something about it. Become a ***conscious eater!***

When you are born again with a conscious mind, you become renewed. No matter how old you are or what your life experiences are, in the self-esteem process, the awakening, there is a need to regroup and retrain yourself. You must become a child again. How do you do that? Through the scriptures, I will try to help you acknowledge the facts and truths that have been with you all the time. Only this time you are awake. You must *"be a doer of the word, and not hearers only, deceiving your own selves. For if any be a hearer of the word and not a doer, he is like unto a man beholding his natural face in a glass: For beholdeth himself, and goeth his way, and straitway forgetteth what manner of man he was. But whoso looketh into the perfect law of liberty, and continueth therein, he being not a forgetful hearer, but a doer of the work, this man shall be blessed in his deed"* (James 1:23–25).

Acknowledgment 1

The fear of the Lord is the beginning of knowledge: but fools despise wisdom and instruction.
Proverbs 1:7

Have you ever known someone who has gone through a traumatic experience, such as a heart attack, kidney failure, diabetes, cancer, car accident, fall, etc.? These traumatic experiences may push the person closer to their consciousness or awakening. People may say to themselves, "If only I could have lived differently, stopped smoking, stopped overeating, stopped drinking, or stopped risky behaviors." Sometimes, through the traumatic experiences, people receive a physical awakening. A physical awakening occurs when one comes to the conclusion of "I want to do right." The statement may be "I am going to do what is right. I am not doing that again." These are good intentions, but are they enough? Why is it that after someone has surgery for a major chronic disease, e.g., heart disease or cancer, and possesses the determination or intentions of doing right, he then goes back to the same lifestyle behaviors, such as smoking, physical inactivity, poor eating habits, etc.? And why is it that someone will have surgery for gastric bypass or stomach stapling, only to go back to the same lifestyle behavior, i.e., overeating, physical inactivity, etc.? One reason is because the good intentions were not accompanied by a spiritual awakening. A spiritual awakening will expand your mind and help you *not* to be closer to your consciousness, but *to be conscious/awake*, making good decisions for yourself.

A good example of a conscious mind is developing a fear of God. In the Old Testament, people were stoned to death for idolatry, blasphemy, lying, adultery, and breaking the Sabbath[1-6]. People who saw the crime and/or the punishment (stoning) were fearful and made a conscious decision not to break God's laws and commandments. (By the way, the laws and commandments were established to provide you with love, peace and joy.) People who kept God's laws knew love. They had love for God, for themselves, and for their neighbor. It was good and it felt good because there are no laws against love.[7]

What if someone loaned you a priceless car and asked you to take care of it until they returned? While they were gone out of town, would you go racing in that car or take it places so that you may be seen in that automobile? The right thing to do is to take care of it; protect it. You should fear the car owner, so that nothing bad happens. Also, you should review the manual to determine how to care for it. Thus, you develop a *fear* of doing the wrong thing (reckless behavior) and you establish a *love* to do the right thing (good behavior).

So, what about you? Are you priceless?

You are a temple of God.[8] You were bought with a price.[9] You are the lost sheep.[10] You are the lost piece of silver.[11] You are the prodigal son.[12] God is calling you to have **fear to do the wrong thing** but **love to do the right thing**. "Work out your own salvation with fear and trembling."[13] Your salvation is priceless. You should fear that you do not follow what is wrong but strive to do what is right. However, God has "not given us the spirit of fear, but of *power* and of *love* and of a *sound mind*."[14] Even so, your fear of God will eventually turn into the knowledge of God—who loves you! Your will to want to do good will overcome the will to want to do wrong (fleshly thoughts/behavior). To go back to your old ways is likened unto a fool. A fool despises wisdom and instruction. Note: "The spirit indeed is willing but the flesh is weak."[15]

Scripture References

1. Deuteronomy 17:2–6
2. Leviticus 24:10–16
3. Deuteronomy 19:15–20
4. John 8:3–5; Deuteronomy 22:22-24
5. Exodus 31:12-17
6. Numbers 15:32–35
7. Galatians 5:22-23
8. 1 Corinthians 3:16–17
9. 1 Corinthians 6: 20
10. Luke 15: 1–7
11. Luke 15: 8–10
12. Luke 15:11–24
13. Philippians 2:12–13
14. 2 Timothy 1:7
15. Matthew 26:41

Acknowledgment 2

This kind can come forth by nothing, but by prayer and fasting.
Mark 9:29

When you acknowledge that there is a problem and it's ailing you, your conscious mind seeks a new role to fix the problem. At first, your conscious mind (MIND) must be acknowledged by your unconscious mind (BODY). Fasting can begin this acknowledgment process. Fasting is one of the worst experiences your body/unconscious mind may encounter: denying yourself of your body's wants and perhaps perceived needs. Denying yourself helps you to reach ground zero—shedding the fleshly motives and desires. This process helps to detach the unconscious mind and its control and gives the rightful owner (conscious mind) the power and leadership role that is so needed for the body.

Prayer and Fasting

A one-day fast is all that is recommended (see Appendix C) to experience the denial process of the selfish you (unconscious mind) and reveal the natural power of the true mind (consciousness). In this fasting process, the conscious mind will develop a role of making right decisions and having more authoritative talks (parent) with the unconscious mind (child). This process is difficult for some, but finding that authoritative voice is necessary because "a double-minded man is unstable in all his ways."[1] Over time, it will take practice. No matter how difficult the process, this is normal! It will take some time and practice but eventually the unconscious mind (child) will look to the conscious mind (parent) for direction and instruction. Eventually, decisions that are made by the unconscious mind (child) will be sound decisions with little effort, if any, from the conscious mind (parent). A sound mind and body is established. This process establishes a meaningful communication relationship that is vital for the mind and body. Nevertheless, communication is the key. Communication between the conscious mind (parent) and the unconscious mind and body (child) are essential. This can be achieved through prayer and fasting.

Prayer is a spiritual communication link between God and you. One recommendation is "And when thou prayest, thou shalt not be as the hypocrites are: for they love to pray standing in the synagogues and in the corners of the street, that they may be seen of men. Verily I say unto you, they have their reward. But thou, when thou prayest, enter into thy closet, and when thou hast shut thy door, pray to thy Father which is in secret, and thy Father which seeth in secret shall reward thee openly."[2]

Fasting is a physical communication link between God, you, and your body. One recommendation is "Moreover when ye fast, be not, as the hypocrites, of a sad countenance: for they disfigure their faces, that they may appear unto men to fast. Verily, I say unto you, they have their reward. But thou, when thou fastest, anoint thine head, and wash thy face, that thou appear not unto men to fast but unto thy Father which is in secret: and thy Father, which seeth in secret, shall reward thee openly."[3]

"Watch and pray, that ye enter not into temptation, the Spirit indeed is willing, but the flesh is weak." Matthew 26:41

Scripture References
1. James 1:8
2. Matthew 6:5–6
3. Matthew 6:16–18

Acknowledgment 3

Whether therefore ye eat, or drink, or whatsoever ye do, do all to the glory of God. 1 Corinthians 10:31

In your awake/conscious state, your body works for you. Your mind can be taught. You can train your mind. Your mind has the power to lead your body to do things that are helpful for you. Sometimes you must fight within your mind to put your body in check. It is a struggle! It is a struggle right now because all children (infant minds) want to test leadership and the parent. This acknowledgment will take more practice and more discipline than any other acknowledgment.

1. When you sit down to eat, are you reading a newspaper, watching the news, or talking?

2. When you are eating, are you chewing, gulping, swallowing your food whole? How many times do you chew before you swallow?

Conscious eating is a physical awareness of bodily functions and the environment during the eating process so that one knows when to stop the process because the body has achieved a level of being comfortably full and obtained enough energy to carry out daily activities to fulfill one's purpose in life.

Conscious eating is a spiritual awareness of God's word as a source of spiritual food. It includes a desire to meditate on God's word that will feed, build and restore a person's mind and body in order to fulfill one's purpose in life.

Essentially, conscious eating is eating with a purpose – a necessity to live. Conscious eating is a necessity to live. It will become a necessity to eat so you can live to do God's will. An example of conscious eating is sitting in a peaceful atmosphere. Experience the eating. Experience every aspect of the environment around you. Look at the food that was prepared for you. See the rich colors, see and feel the texture, smell the aroma. Try a strawberry. See the love. Appreciate God's love that went into making that strawberry for you. This is an experience you do not want to miss! This conscious eating is eating to live.

When you have found your purpose in life and you are actually living with a purpose, sometimes eating becomes secondary. Your purpose for living may become so overwhelming that you forget to eat. You may forget the necessities of food until the true hunger pang rings the bell. "I am hungry, and I can't function without food," says the body. Like a car, the body cannot operate properly without fuel, namely food. In essence, you give the body the fuel it needs to keep on moving and living the purpose for which it was created. You eat to *live!*

Occasional pleasure eating is okay, as long as the conscious mind is aware of it. However, when pleasurable eating is done unconsciously, it is dangerous and should be avoided at all cost.

In the past, when soda pop was consumed, six ounces was an individual serving. This one six-ounce soda was consumed as a treat, usually because people could not afford more of it or it was a pleasure to drink soda pop on weekends or once a month (sparingly). Now vending machines are selling twenty-ounce sodas (more than three times the amount sold years ago). Individuals consume one twenty-ounce soda a day or as much as six times a day or a twelve-pack a day. When excess soda is consumed, who is making this decision: the conscious mind (parent) or the unconscious mind (child)?

Would you give a two-year-old a soda every day? Would you give a two-year-old a six pack of soda every day? Would you allow a child to make parental decisions? The conscious mind (parent) needs to communicate to the unconscious mind (child). This is to say that pleasurable eating should be used solely as a treat and you must ask what and how much of a food item should be eaten. The parent sets the limits on how much of this pleasurable food is allowed for that day, that month, or that year.

In any case, whether you are eating to live or eating for pleasure, do it to the glory of God.

Acknowledgment 4

**Thou shalt love the Lord thy God with all thy heart,
and with all thy soul, and with all thy mind
… Thou shalt love thy neighbor as thyself.
Matthew 22:37–39.**

When you put God first, the unconscious mind (self) has no more room. Selfish deeds, such as buying a combo meal, will become apparent as selfishness and greed, and overeating may result. Taking the time to sit down to overeat is a selfish act and physically abusive to a temple of God. This act will not allow the conscious mind to fully serve God.

When you realize that God has not given you a spirit of fear but of power and of love and of a sound mind, then you are able to realize the greatest commandments of all: "Thou shalt love the Lord thy God with all thy heart, and with all thy soul, and with all thy mind … Thou shalt love thy neighbor as thyself."

As your mind and body reach ground zero and begin to build up in a concerted effort, a balance is established. In addition, every part of your being knows its role. Your spiritual mind is stronger, willing and able, and the flesh truly is weakened, humbled, and seeking direction from the mind (parent).

In James 3, the tongue is described as a member of the body that defileth the whole body. Who can tame the tongue—an unruly evil full of deadly poison? James goes on to say that a horse, a ship, and beasts are able to be tamed by man. Yet the tongue, a small member of the body, is not able to be tamed, and proceeds to defile the whole body.[1] How can this be?

How is it that a doctor can do surgery to save lives, yet smoke cigarettes? How is it that a dietitian can counsel on nutrition, yet be overweight? How is it that a teacher can teach economics or math, yet files for bankruptcy? How is it that a person has been diagnosed with diabetes, yet continues to eat fried foods and sweets? How is it that a person can be overweight, yet continue to consume desserts and snacks and not exercise?

How is it that a child can do wrong, yet the parents not correct them? *Wake up! Wake up!*

"Doth a fountain send forth at the same place sweet water and bitter? Can the fig tree, my brethren, bear olive berries? Either a vine, figs? So can no fountain both yield salt water and fresh."[1]

When the whole body is turned around—*turned* around from unconscious living and in unison with self—a sound mind and body establishes an awareness of self and surroundings. Your purpose then becomes clear to love God with all your heart, mind, and soul, and to love thy neighbor as thyself. Your world: God, you, and your neighbor are one; establishing God's Kingdom because His Kingdom lives within you.[2]

Scripture References
1. James 3:11–12
2. Luke 17:21

Acknowledgment 5

Walk in the Spirit, and ye shall not fulfil the lust of the flesh. Galatians 5:16.

Walk is an action word. Do it, w-a-l-k! Do it, w-a-l-k!

Physical activity or exercise is believed to be healthful to the body by many experts and lay people. When you walk in God's creation, you see all of His love, mercies, and blessings everywhere. How can you see it sitting in front of the television? How can you see it in the house? How can you feel or smell it on the computer? Embrace it! God's creation is here!

At least once a week, take a moment out of your busy schedule to embrace the Earth, the creation that God has prepared for you. Take a walk; go to the park or zoo; swim; watch children at play; observe the ants and birds; look at the clear blue sky or clouds; watch the rising or setting of the sun; see the different shapes and sizes of trees. Embrace it! Enjoy it!

When you walk in the Spirit, you see God's creation, including you, the conscious mind, leading and guiding the unconscious mind and body. In order to have a sound mind,[1] you cannot serve two masters.[2] You must worship God in Spirit and Truth.[3] There is no room or time for an unstable mind, the selfish me—the lust of the flesh.

Scripture References
1. 2 Timothy 1:7
2. Luke 16:13
3. John 4:23–24

Acknowledgment 6

Blessed are the poor in Spirit for theirs is the kingdom of heaven. Matthew 5:3.

How can you be blessed when you are *poor in spirit?* Good question. You are *poor in spirit* if you are unconscious and allow the fleshly body and lusts to rule you—the conscious mind.

Arise and walk! Arise and walk!

Now that you are conscious of your poor spirit, do something about it. Your conscious mind—your *spirit*—needs that still, *small* voice[1] to be a *big* voice leading and guiding you into all truth. When you are ready to stand up and make right decisions for the body, everything else will fall into place. Your body is a temple of God and His Spirit dwells in you.[2] God said, "I will put a new spirit within you; that they may walk in my statutes, ordinances, and do them: and they shall be my people, and I will be their God."[3]

In essence, "man shall not live by bread alone, but by every word of God."[4] For the words that God speaks to you, "they are spirit, they are life." [5] Eat God's word daily, to build up your spirit being. God's Word is spiritual food for the soul—the spiritual mind—the conscious mind. A true spiritual awakening gives you the will to do what is right; you no longer want to be poor in spirit but rich in spirit. You want to feed on God's Word to build up the unseen thing—the mind. Also, you recognize that overeating clouds the mind and is the lust of the flesh, which is an enmity of God and your purpose in life.

Whether it's spiritual or physical eating, you want to do what is right. When you recognize your spiritual deficiencies and make a conscious effort to obtain spiritual food and walk in His ways, then God's kingdom becomes a part of you and lives in you.[6] The parable about the prodigal son is a good example.[7]

Scripture References

1. 1 Kings 19:9-12
2. 1 Corinthians 3:16; 6:19
3. Ezekiel 11:19–20; 37:23
4. Luke 4:4
5. John 6:63
6. Luke 17:21
7. Luke 15:11-24

Acknowledgment 7

Blessed are they which do hunger and thirst after Righteousness: for they shall be filled. Matthew 5:6.

Have you ever hungered for something? Or craved something you have not had in a long time? Maybe it's a favorite dish at Thanksgiving; or your aunt's favorite dish; or your favorite restaurant foods. All of these are images you have planted in your mind. These images or smells pop up occasionally. This memory bank of special food—*treats*—provides you with pleasure. Pleasure is good, indeed. But is it the right type of pleasure for your body? If it is not, have a groundbreaking ceremony for your mind. Start tilling the mind and sift through those images.

Your taste buds work for you—the conscious mind. They can be changed. Change them. Teach your unconscious mind (body) to crave and hunger after vegetables and fruits, water, low-fat calcium-rich foods, etc. When you try new recipes or foods, slow down and taste the food for the first time. Your taste buds will eventually change for the better. You will enjoy whole grain products and the fullness it brings your body; you will enjoy the juice from an orange rather than orange juice; you will savor after a natural smoothie rather than ice cream; you will crave water in the middle of the night for cleansing and fullness, rather than a snack that is rich in calories and fat. Replace the old memories of foods you believed your body craved with foods and drinks you know are good for your body.

Ultimately, God's Word is your spiritual food. Jesus said that He is the bread of life and the water that He provides, no man will thirst again.[1] The water that He gives "shall be in him a well of water springing up into everlasting life."[2] God's Word is soul food that keeps your mind on track. Positive thoughts begin to form, and positive actions begin to play out in one's life. Your life's purpose begins to be fulfilled.

Man shall not live by bread alone but by every
word that proceedeth out of the mouth of God.[3]

Scripture References
1. John 6:35–58
2. John 4:13–14
3. Matthew 4:4

Acknowledgment 8

Blessed are the pure in heart: for they shall see God. Matthew 5:8

When you have a stable mind and body in righteousness, you have a pure heart. Your pure heart allows the conscious mind to be in tune with God. This communion with God allows you to be humble as a child,[1] knowing that hearing His voice and following God, He will take care of all of your needs, including food and drink.[2] Your thoughts are not overwhelmed with food or your next meal. "Therefore, take no thought, saying, *What shall we eat? or What shall we drink? or Wherewithal shall we be clothed?* ... But seek first the Kingdom of God, and His righteousness; and all these things shall be added unto you."[3]

Children are innocent and pure. They seek their parents' advice, to lead and guide them to do what is right. We are God's children[4] - His sheep that hear his voice.[5] Having a pure heart allows God to lead you. "Suffer the little children to come unto ME, and forbid them not: *for such is the kingdom of God. Verily I say unto you. Whosoever shall not receive the kingdom of God as a little child, he shall not enter therein.*"[6]

"For if ye live after the flesh, ye shall die: but if ye through the Spirit do mortify the deeds of the body, ye shall live. For as many as are led by the Spirit of God, they are the sons of God. For ye have not received the spirit of bondage again to fear, but ye have received the Spirit of adoption, whereby we cry, Abba, Father."[7]

Scripture References

1. Matthew 18:3–4
2. John 10:11, 14, 27
3. Matthew 6:31, 33
4. Galatians 4:5-7; Revelation 21:7
5. John 10:1-4, 27
6. Mark 10:14, 15
7. Romans 8:13–15

Chapter 2
Truths

The truth shall set you free!

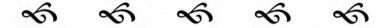

Parents teach children how to eat. Through their life experiences and wisdom, they teach children eating habits at an early age. Some of these teachings stem from traditions and environment. They are simple statements, ideas or instructions that a parent may have used to guide a child or teenager in eating or drinking. These statements are meant to be a guide for retraining your thought process and behavior in relations to food. The Truth statements or other parts of this book have not been evaluated by the Food and Drug Administration or the United States Department of Agriculture.

The Truth statements mentioned in this section may be familiar or unfamiliar, depending on your generation. You may have heard these truths as a child or teenager. Just as you can always count on your parents or a good friend to tell you the truth, now you (Parent—conscious mind) may acknowledge these Truth statements and establish them as your eating habits. Be a *doer* and not a hearer only.

Note: The Truth statements are drawn from the author's life experiences.

In each truth, there is a model statement. Say them out loud! Meditate on them. Create new ones if needed. Whatever the case may be, change your thought process. *Speak* is an action word. Speak out loud as you open the refrigerator, as you go to the grocery store, as you order your food in a restaurant, as you prepare your food for your family or yourself. Yes, speak even when temptations come, because they will come. (James 1:14) Change your thought process and life patterns! You can do this!

Truth 1
You are what you eat.

Your spiritual and physical body tells a lot about who you are. Meditating on scriptures loaded with instruction, advice, and wisdom helps the spiritual body to grow, repair, and restore. Consuming foods loaded with nutrients needed for the body helps the body to grow, repair, and restore. Ask yourself. "What am I?" Are you a healthy individual both spiritually and physically?

Statement: You are what you eat! You are what you eat!

Truth 2
Eat all of your vegetables and fruits.

Vegetables and fruits offer a lot of vitamins, minerals, and fiber that are needed by the body. However, the unconscious body wants to rebel and pursue the cruise-control attitude and eat everything but vegetables and fruits. Taste buds can change. Thus, communication becomes essential between the mind and the body. Remember, the body and all its members, including the taste buds, work for you—the conscious mind. The parent (conscious mind) needs to encourage and talk to their child (unconscious body) daily to get the necessary response and outcome from the child.

Statement: Tell yourself (unconscious body—child) you need more vegetables and fruits. "Eat more vegetables and fruits." Repeat it. "Vegetables and fruits are good for you."

Truth 3
Don't eat too much or your tummy will hurt!

Avoid distractions, such as television, reading, and talking. The fewer distractions, the more you can focus on the child (unconscious body) to see how much you have eaten. Also, you can listen to the child (body), because the body communicates and cues you when you are full. If the child is not monitored, chances are, he will do something unnoticeable through an autopilot/cruise-control action. Note: The child does not want to harm themselves but without proper guidance and protection they are liable to make unconscious decisions that may cause them harm. Thus, an autopilot action, such as unconscious eating may harm you by causing you to overeat. As a result, you FEEL BAD.

Practice eating until you are *"comfortably full,"* not stuffed! When you are finished eating, get up from the table and do something else. Just push away from the table. Your need for food has been satisfied. Now do other activities in your life: chores, hobbies, conversation in the living room, take out the garbage, watch the news or your favorite television program, read a book, read to your children, help your children with their homework, walk in nature or your neighborhood, visit with a neighbor, write a letter, phone a friend, attend a support group meeting, workout at the gym or do other activities that fulfill your specific purpose in this lifetime.

Statement: Tell yourself—"Your tummy will hurt if you eat too much of _____." Eat because it is a necessity to live. Practice eating until you are comfortably full, not stuffed.

Truth 4
Eat to live and not live to eat.

How many times have you gotten up in the morning and you are looking for something to eat? Sometimes you can't even wash your face or brush your teeth without eating or drinking something first. Are you living to eat?

At work around noontime, do you break for lunch and eat because it's noon? Are you truly hungry? Your body has the same cues as a baby when he or she cries for food. Not many of us have the flexibility during a workday to eat sporadically on a flexible schedule, but if you schedule your meals appropriately, just like a baby starts to cry every three to four hours and the parent is prepared to breast- or bottle-feed them, your body will follow a similar pattern. After some consideration of your body's need, your body will provide cues of "I am hungry." As a parent (mind), you should have meals or snacks prepared and ready for your child (body). The job for the conscious mind is to be the parent who is prepared to feed that child (unconscious body) the healthy foods it needs to live. Your body will begin to look for directions from the mind to eat to live and not live to eat. The parent should not wait until extreme hunger—which may result in overeating, but slight hunger—to feed the body healthy foods to live longer, healthier, and stronger. As a result, your foods will be a source of fuel or energy the body needs to fulfill your purpose in life.

Statement: I will listen to the body for true cues of hunger. (You will know the hunger cues from your fasting experience at ground zero.) Eat to live and not live to eat.

Truth 5
Sit down to eat.

We live in a fast-paced world with microwave ovens, fast foods, etc. So many times we are eating in our cars, on the way to work or home. We are sipping on a soft drink or coffee on our way to the next chore, errand, or meeting. We need to slow down and pay attention to the child (unconscious body) who needs you, the parent (conscious mind). The child cannot raise itself and needs attention and support. We see it all the time, when a single parent leaves his or her oldest child to raise the younger children. Although this is possible, it is not ideal. A parent is required to give the emotional and physical support the child needs and craves. As a parent, you need to slow down and see the importance of eating in a peaceful atmosphere. Set the stage of eating for yourself as if you invited a friend or family member to have dinner at your house. Eating by yourself or with family should be a pleasant experience, and not rushed. Watch yourself eat. Watch yourself breathe while you eat. Enjoy the experience! Be thankful for the food you have and briefly meditate on those who live daily without food. Don't take food for granted! God provided food for you to eat and enjoy.

Statement: Relax; enjoy the food that was prepared just for you. Sit down to eat!

Truth 6
Chew your food.

If you watch a toddler eat, you will notice something. A lot of times, children eat food without chewing properly, so the parent has to remind them to chew their food. As a child, you may have heard "Chew your food 32 times before swallowing." Whether it is more or less than 32 times, when you properly chew your food, your body does not have to work as hard. Your body actually smiles and thanks you, the parent (conscious mind). Your teeth are there for a reason, not for a brighter smile (though this is nice). Your teeth are there to help you chew so your food is properly digested. Use your teeth; they are working for you (conscious mind). When you don't chew appropriately, your teeth are working for the unconscious mind. Have you ever swallowed some food whole by mistake? What happened? Your throat and/or stomach may have felt some pain or discomfort indicating that you did not chew your food properly. As a result, your stomach had to work harder.

Statement: I have teeth; they are sharp and capable of chewing. I **must use** my teeth to digest my food properly. Chew your food.

Truth 7
Your skin looks terrible; stop drinking all that soda. Drink water!

As a teenager, your mother, aunt, or other relatives saw that you were not only going through puberty but started this unconscious behavior of drinking too many sodas or soft drinks or other things not healthy for you. Water is essential for the body. The body needs water daily. Our bodies are made up of 70 to 80 percent water. We need water to replenish and flush out toxins daily. Water can do this. Kidneys crave water in order to do their job properly. Do you take long, warm baths? Why? Maybe it is for pleasure, but also to get clean. Do you drink fewer than three glasses of water a day? Why? Three glasses will certainly make your kidneys work harder. Also, it would be difficult to take a thorough bath or shower with less than three glasses of water. Drinking six to eight glasses a day is similar to that nice long shower you take on the outside of the body. Drink six to eight glasses of water a day for an internal body bath. Thank God for providing clean and fresh water for you.

Statement: I need water to help my kidneys. I need a good shower on the inside of my body. Drink six to twelve glasses of water a day. (Depending on your body size, you may need more or less water per day)

Truth 8
Don't eat late at night.

Many restaurants are open 24 hours or advertise late hours on certain days. This is happy hour for the unconscious body (child) and ludicrous for the conscious mind (parent). Would you allow your child to eat a burger, fries, and soft drink at midnight? Late at night, the conscious mind/parent should be telling the unconscious body/child to go to sleep and get rest. However, during these crucial hours when the digestive system and other bodily systems need their rest, the unconscious body (child) defies authority just like a teenager would with new freedom. However, if you "Train up a child in the way he should go: and when he is old, he will not depart from it." (Proverbs 22:6) Nighttime eating is hazardous to your health. Your body has to work harder when it should be resting. Oftentimes, extra calories are consumed that the body does not need or burn during the night.

Statement: Nighttime hours are for relaxing, winding down, and resting. Go to bed and let your body do what it does best at night—rest—not eat.

Truth 9
Drink your milk!

Milk has many useful properties for the body. Milk has protein, calcium, Vitamin A, Vitamin D, and other nutrients. Recently, milk and other calcium-rich products are noted to help people to maintain or lose weight. Unfortunately, very few people drink milk. There is a major decline in milk consumption over the years among the child and adolescent population, and probably for the adult population too. If you are unable to drink milk, try a few suggestions:

1. Drink a small amount of milk with your meals and gradually increase your consumption, if you are able to tolerate it.
2. Consume low-fat yogurt and/or cheese.
3. Consume calcium-rich foods and/or drinks i.e., fortified cereals and juices, almonds, salmon with bones, soy milk and cheese, goat's milk, and greens.
4. Ask your doctor for more information on dietary supplements if necessary.

Statement: I will make a conscious effort to include a minimum of two servings of low-fat calcium-rich products every day. If I am unsuccessful, I will talk to my healthcare provider for an appropriate type and amount of dietary supplement for me. Note: Too much Calcium may cause constipation and other problems.

Truth 10
Eat your foods before you drink your juice.

Many parents have strong beliefs that a child who drinks his juice before eating will spoil his appetite. Overtime if a child consumes juice and juice drinks prior to their meals they may consume excess amount of calories and not consume high nutrient dense foods needed for a crucial growth period. A parent's ideal child would consume all the healthy foods prepared for him, and juice would be a treat after the meal; maybe on weekends or once a month. Also, if all the healthy foods are consumed, very little juice is needed to satisfy the total nutrients needed by the body. Also, there would be less room in the tummy to consume too much juice or juice drink.

Another belief is that drinks should be consumed an hour before or two hours after a meal for better digestion. Drinking with a meal or before or after is a decision that should be made by the parent. You (conscious mind) decide what's best for your child.

Statement: Your food is your main source of energy, vitamins, minerals, and fiber for the body. Drink juice as a treat.

Truth 11
Enough is Enough!

Going to an all-you-can-eat buffet is good for the unconscious mind. It is a food playground. A child (unconscious body) can run wild without any rules. When people leave such restaurants, they leave uncomfortable: loosening their pants, sleepy, unable to move, intoxicated with food. All of this is done with the mindset of "getting my money's worth" while causing the body physical harm. Your unconscious body fooled you again to believe it is mature enough to make right decisions for you. Like a teenager, your body makes you believe it can handle this type of freedom and decision-making. Big mistake. Most teenagers (unconscious body) have not reached the level of maturity to make conscious decisions about food intake. So the conscious mind must be in control. Control is to say, "No, we cannot go to the food playground (all-you-can-eat restaurant), because you don't know how to act." Or the conscious mind needs to say, "When we get to the food playground, I will tell you when enough is enough."

Have you experienced comfortably full? *This takes practice.* Comfortably full is when your body has eaten enough for necessity and sustainability to live.

A new mindset of "Enough is Enough" with the pain and agony of being overfed—physical abuse: coughing, bloating, sluggish, impaired mental capabilities will be established.

Try three ounces of meat or beans, two ounces of grains, one-half cup of vegetable, one-half cup of fruit, and one cup of milk or alternative food or drink for a dinner meal. Eat until your body becomes comfortably full. This means you must chew your food well, sit down to eat your vegetables and fruits, and consume calcium rich products. All of this should take

15 - 30 minutes. Eventually, your body will send cues to the mind to say, "I am full. Stop eating!" You are comfortably full. As a result, 'Enough is Enough' is fulfilled in your thoughts and actions!

Statement: Enough is Enough!

Truth 12
Bonus
Go outside and play!

Do you have good memories of being outside until the mosquitoes started to bite you? But then you went outside the next day, even with all the mosquito bites. Fun is fun. Children know how to have fun. Have you bought several toys for a child, only to notice that they played with the box the toy came in or used your pots and pans for toys? Children know how to have fun. It's very simple—just do whatever. Pillow fights, tickling, hide and seek, laughing, telling jokes, jumping (hopscotch and jump rope), snowball fights, walking in the rain without shoes, watching a sunset or a rainbow, dancing, swimming, whatever! Do it. It will change your life.

Statement: Go outside and play! (Say it like your mom would say it! Smile.)

CHAPTER 3
Reflections

What do you see?

Many people like to look in the mirror to see him or herself. Have you observed a baby looking into a mirror? Most of them laugh. Laughing at yourself is good. This is the beginning of self-awareness. When children see themselves for the first time in the mirror, many of them laugh because they become aware of the being that exists—"That's me!" Also, when they walk for the first time, another realization occurs and they may laugh because once again they realize "It's me. My legs, my muscles are doing that thing! Walking!" This self-awareness is a new thing, and when you see your reflection for the first time, sometimes you cannot help but to laugh at yourself!

Other times, you may not laugh at your reflection. Have you ever taken a 360-degree look at yourself? Really? Sometimes people will shy away from taking a picture because of what they may see. Even with a camera view of themselves, some people may become sad, because the picture that was captured by the camera is not the person they thought they would see. The picture may show the reality of the 10, 20, 30 pounds that were gained in the face, arms, and everywhere else on the body. The child knew about it because larger clothes were bought and worn to cover up evidence, but the parent was obviously asleep when all this occurred. When a digital camera instantly shows the picture of you—then the initial shock takes place, such as "Look at my face" or "Boy, do I look overweight!" Through this camera view, you may see a true reflection, and you get the parent's awareness. This is similar to a child who brings home a bad report card and the parent asks, "How did this happen?"

"How did *this* happen to me? How did I gain so much weight?"

Think back! An example is when the fall and winter holidays were approaching. Everyone was having parties and gatherings, and the peer pressure was overwhelming. It became so overwhelming that the parent never set any guidelines and allowed the child to have a few treats. However, the child nagged and nagged until treats became a regular activity. So much nagging (constant thoughts, reasoning, self talk about food) occurred that a dessert and treat throughout the day became a normal routine. It was a food playground, week after week then day after day. Yet something strange happened: there were no more holidays, but the child has been in control for several days, weeks, and months. It has not been easy for the child to relinquish the power back to the parent, who has been asleep throughout the holidays and months afterward. "The food playground feels good; who needs structure?" is the child's self-talk. And the parent listens.

Press the FORWARD button!

Someone is taking a picture of *you* with a digital camera. (Be reminded the child does not want to take the picture—the evidence is too great.) What is your reflection? You are what you eat!

Sometimes when parents dress their child, they see a reflection of themselves. They try to make corrections wherever necessary, such as washing their face, brushing their teeth, combing their hair, tucking in their shirt, pulling up their pants, putting the shoes on the right foot.

Now look into the mirror and what do you see? If not a mirror, pretend there are video cameras in your kitchen window or on the wall. What will the mirror reflect or camera capture on tape? Will it capture repeated times when you went to the kitchen cabinet or refrigerator for food or a snack or drink? Will it capture you eating late at night when you should be in bed asleep? Will it reflect a person watching a TV commercial only to trigger something in the mind that makes you want to snack on food when you are not hungry? Will it capture you going to get some gas for the car and picking up a candy bar and soda *just because?* Just because ... You are unconscious when you are making these decisions. You are not considering what is good and right for the body.

For example, one day I entered a restaurant on my lunch break. I had great intentions of getting a chicken sandwich and a salad. I did not need a diet soda, because I had a diet soda in the office refrigerator. I reminded myself of the soda even before I left the office by saying "I don't need a soda with my meal, because I will have it when I return to the office." Also, I decided that I would not have a drink with my meal. One, I was trying to save money by buying drinks in bulk, and two I was trying to save money by not buying a drink in a combo meal.

When I went into the restaurant, I ordered a chicken sandwich and a salad. The cashier said, "Would you like to have a combo?"

I said, "Is that cheaper?"

She said, "Yes."

Immediately, I said, "Yes, I will have a combo." I sat down to eat and laughed at myself (self-awareness). That child (unconscious mind) made the decision at the counter and tried to reason that it's cheaper to buy a combo. The parent (conscious mind) sat back and paid for it without a fight. As I began to eat my meal, I ate my sandwich and drank half of my soda and saved my salad for the next day.

Although I allowed the transaction of the combo meal to occur, I did not have to sit there to consume the whole meal, which was too much for me. So with love, I took extra precautions to sit down, eat, and chew my food slowly. I listened to my body, and I noticed when I became comfortably full. The drink was my treat, so I only allowed myself to drink half of it. The salad was good for me, but it was too much at this time. I was comfortably full. I had to say enough is enough. Later I felt good both mentally and physically. It **FEELS GOOD** to **FEEL GOOD**. The parent was back in control.

Every day for the next week, look for instances when your conscious mind and unconscious mind communicate, especially about decisions with food. When you see yourself, determine who is making the decision. Is it the parent (mind) or the child (body) making the decisions? Once you mentally see the reflections of yourself in the mirror, camera make the necessary corrections with love.

Sunday   Date _____
Conscious Mind (Parent)

_____
_____
_____
_____

Unconscious Mind (Child)

_____
_____
_____
_____

Monday   Date _____
Conscious Mind (Parent)

_____
_____
_____
_____

Unconscious Mind (Child)

_____
_____
_____
_____

Tuesday   Date _____
Conscious Mind (Parent)

_____
_____
_____
_____

Unconscious Mind (Child)

_____
_____

Wednesday   Date _____
Conscious Mind (Parent)

_____
_____
_____
_____
_____

Unconscious Mind (Child)

_____
_____
_____
_____
_____

Thursday   Date _____
Conscious Mind (Parent)

_____
_____
_____
_____
_____

Unconscious Mind (Child)

_____
_____
_____
_____
_____

Friday   Date _____
Conscious Mind (Parent)

_____
_____
_____
_____
_____
_____
_____

Unconscious Mind (Child)

_____

_____

_____

_____

_____

Saturday   Date _____
Conscious Mind (Parent)

_____

_____

_____

_____

_____

Unconscious Mind (Child)

_____

_____

_____

_____

_____

Now consider the changes you will make and list them (This will become part of your Track Record):

_____

_____

_____

_____

_____

_____

_____

_____

Oftentimes, children are observant and honest. Parents may need to quiet them so their honesty does not offend anybody. However, what children see and say may be innocent and honest.

I encourage you to look around your environment and be conscious, especially when it comes to you and your neighbor's health. Through my eyes, the reflections that I see are:

- A generation of children who will not live past 30 years of age due to chronic illnesses and diseases
- Two young black men practicing walking with sticks to guide them down the street because they are blind; it is possible that they have recently become blind due to a chronic disease such as diabetes
- New dialysis centers being built in neighborhoods
- Native children who are overweight and suffering from diabetes
- Elementary students who cannot run because of excess weight and joint problems
- Children who eat unconsciously in front of the television or computer
- Children who eat chips and drink soda for breakfast before the bus picks them up
- Health food store manager and staff who are overweight and sell weight loss products
- A generation of children who do not know how to ride a bike
- Restaurant ads that promote late-night eating
- Whole communities with fast food restaurants, gas stations, liquor and corner stores filled with low nutrient - high dense foods and limited fresh or high nutrient foods
- A black man who died at 33 years of age because of kidney failure due to uncontrolled blood pressure
- Children who eat any- and everything at anytime—no structure or guidance
- Children who consume soda, chips, and candies instead of school breakfast and lunch
- A four-year-old black male with high blood pressure
- Restaurant ads that promote the biggest burger for the money
- Preteen girls who are shaped like women and wearing women-sized clothes

- Communities with grocery stores with limited choices of fresh, appealing and healthy foods at a reasonable price
- Health professionals who cannot reach the middle-aged black man to lose excess weight –Prevention
- Specialty treatment centers and hospitals that are marketed on billboards, radios, and television stations. -Treatment
- Overweight parents and overweight children
- Middle-aged people carrying breathing machines to do their daily chores
- Mothers who are overworked, stressed, and may not have time or desire to prepare a decent meal for their family and fast food is a staple for the family diet
- Middle-aged overweight people with walking sticks and walkers
- People who live in rural areas with limited access to recreational activities
- Young people who avoid going to the movies because they fear they will not fit in the theater seats
- A forty-year-old black male with uncontrolled diabetes that resulted in nerve damage in his feet. He later filed for disability because he could no longer work due to excruciating pain while walking and doing daily chores
- People who avoid walking because of unsafe neighborhoods due to crime, unleashed dogs, etc.
- A 36 year old black man newly diagnosed with kidney disease and needing dialysis
- Sales for medications are steadily increasing and pharmacy stores are within miles of each other including in your local grocery stores
- A Caucasian mother who is not concerned about her young son's overweight status because she believes in his future of being the next famous football player
- Overweight single black man dies because of diabetes complications at 32 years of age
- Children walking with a limp because their joints are in pain due to excess weight
- Overweight may be seen as a status symbol of good health and wealth in some cultures

- Middle-aged people living in nursing homes whose limbs were amputated and they are in wheelchairs
- Men who are diagnosed with breast cancer
- People who are heavy consumers of quick fixes for weight loss, only to lose the weight and regain it with additional pounds
- Food used as a drug in some cases similar to smoking cigarettes, and drinking alcohol, yet not given the same consideration when it comes to prevention or treatment
- Young people riding motorized grocery carts to shop because they are unable to walk due to excess weight
- Healthcare cost that are constantly rising, but very few people ask "Why is this happening?" or "How can we prevent it?" (Just as an Unconscious Parent, we find ways to pay for the health care costs – Treatment versus dealing with accountability and prevention as a Conscious Parent)
- Overweight 32 year black woman dies because of diabetes complications. Before she died, she was in a wheel chair because her legs were amputated.
- Children with bulging shoes because of their limp walk and large feet.
- Overweight adults and children who have difficulties with tying their shoes.
- Airline companies that require overweight people to purchase two plane tickets because extra seating in not available and they cannot sit in one seat comfortably
- Children who do not consume enough Calcium and Vitamin D and potentially have a high risk of fragile bones and teeth before they reach middle age
- People less than fifty years of age in the obituary section of the newspaper

What do you see around you?

_____

_____

_____

_____

_____

_____

_____

_____

_____

_____

_____

_____

_____

_____

_____

_____

_____

_____

_____

_____

_____

_____

_____

_____

_____

_____

_____

_____

_____

_____

_____

_____

CHAPTER 4
Who Is Knocking at the Door?

Open Your Mind and Body

A long time ago, my brother and I would hear the doorbell ring and see some people dressed up at the door. Peeping through the curtains, we would duck and dodge the door and their conversation. The people we avoided were from a religious organization. Over the years, I have developed an acceptance of various religions, belief systems, values, etc. Having an open mind, I have found many treasures in God's Kingdom. I know there is an awesome God, a Higher Power that exists, and you see evidence of His existence every day—in people, in nature, in situations, etc.

God is LOVE.[1] God is the Alpha and Omega. God is the First and the Last.[2] God is Everything. God is ALL.[3]

Healthy conversations about God are good. So many times, we are divided because of particular religious beliefs and systems, and we forget the basics of loving God with all of your heart, mind, and soul, and loving your neighbor as yourself. Yes, we ought to "rightly divide the word of truth."[4] However, even knowledge without charity is nothing.[5] Whenever two or more are gathered in His name, He is there also.[6] While man has established religion based on his present knowledge of God, it is all a heavenly experience in these earthly bodies if you know your purpose in life. You can seize the opportunity to expand your mind and broaden your spiritual horizons by living consciously. Sophisticated barriers keep us from these special experiences. Be encouraged to discuss God and His creation with others in love. We are all His children, His creation. We make up the Body of Christ.[7] We cannot continue to say we love God who we do not see and hate our neighbor who we see every day.[8]

Wake up! Arise, walk and talk in the spirit. I beseech you, brothers and sisters, do not close your ears and your eyes. Open up the door to your heart that you may be healed.

"Go unto this people and say, Hearing ye shall hear and shall not understand. And seeing ye shall see, and not perceive. For the heart of this people is waxed gross, and their ears are dull of hearing, and their eyes have they closed, lest they should see with their eyes, and understand with their heart, and should be converted and I should heal them."[9]

"Behold, I stand at the DOOR and KNOCK: if any man hear my voice; and open the door, I will come into him and will SUP with him, and he with me. To him that OVERCOMETH will I grant to sit with ME in my throne, even as I also OVERCAME, and am set down with my Father in His throne. He that hath an ear, let him hear what the SPIRIT saith unto the churches."[10]

Whether it's God speaking to you through His Word or a casual conversation about God with a friend or stranger, don't duck and dodge the great opportunities to listen to that still small voice that will guide you in your daily walk, including your eating habits. Enjoy the healthy conversations about God with a friend or stranger. It will strengthen your faith or you may encourage someone else. Open the door to your heart and commune with God and share with others.

Who is knocking at the door to your heart?

Scripture References

1. 1 John 4:16
2. Revelation 1:11
3. Colossians 3:11
4. 2 Timothy 2:15
5. 1 Corinthians 13:2
6. Matthew 18:20
7. 1 Corinthians 12:12–31
8. 1 John 4:20–21
9. Acts 28:26-27; Isaiah 6:9-10
10. Revelation 3:20-22

PART 2:
KNOWLEDGE
PLANT THE SEEDS

CHAPTER 5
Build Up Your Mind!

The Unseen Thing

You know that *something* exists to allow the sun to rise every morning. That *something* is unseen. Some people call that existence God, a Higher Power, Jehovah, Jesus, and many other names. Whatever that spiritual existence is to you—tap into it! This is your source of spiritual power—an unseen force that helps you to cope with those physical challenges. Your spiritual connection is your source of power to overcome the temptations of the flesh. If you have a poor connection (poor in spirit) and your challenges with food are difficult, then recognize it and do something about it. If you have a strong spiritual connection, then you can resist the temptations and they shall flee from you. Build up the unseen thing by eating spiritual food—change your thought process and hunger and thirst after righteousness.

What is your purpose in this life?

Many of us have a ball-and-chain lifestyle when it comes to food—"a live-to-eat mentality." For example, we may complete a major project at work, so our minds and bodies may say, "Let's splurge at an all-you-can-eat restaurant to celebrate." Our child becomes so accustomed to having treats or special-occasion eating periods—that these treats and special occasions become *daily*. The body is telling the mind what to do instead of the mind telling the body what to do. Oftentimes there is a disconnect and too many voices or members of the body are saying and doing things that are inappropriate for the body. This is where the lust of the flesh is powerful and the mind/parent is sitting in the corner, not doing or saying anything, when in actuality, the parent (mind) has the biggest voice of all the members. How do you empower the mind?

Ask yourself, "What is my purpose in life?" What do you plan to do with your life tomorrow, next week, next month, next year, in five or ten years? When you have a purpose, you have goals and plans to reach those goals. Allow your body to work for you.

For example, do you want to be a nurse to help people? Then ask yourself, "What am I doing to obtain a nursing degree?" Do you want to be a small-business owner? What steps have you taken to make this happen? Before you retired, what was "it" that you wanted to do when you retired? Are you doing those things? Are you living with a purpose, even though you are not working? Volunteering at a hospital, nursing home, or daycare may be your purpose. Perhaps it's to help someone? When you focus on your life purpose—your ball and chain—your burden of food is lifted. Jesus said, "Come unto me all ye that labour and are heavy laden and I will give you rest."[1]

Take a look at your life. Are you a caregiver for everyone else except for *yourself*? If so, you must first take care of yourself before you can help others, not the opposite. Many people do a good job in taking care of others in their family and at work. We take pride in seeing others succeed, but when it comes to ourselves, we take a back seat and are unconscious of the lifestyle we are living while helping others.

If you have ever flown on a plane, the stewardess gives you specific instructions about assisting a young child in a flight emergency. They instruct you to put on your breathing mask first, then begin to assist others. Think about it. Why is this? If you are not functioning or unconscious, then you can't possibly begin to help others. If the child has a mask on and you faint, can the child help you? No. You must first learn to help yourself so that you can be a good vessel or mentor to help others.

Although this is not a weight-loss book, are you overweight? Do your clothes fit snugly? Do you want to lose weight and be at a comfortable and healthy weight for your body? What steps are you taking to take care of your body? Is losing five pounds per month for the next six months your goal? Regardless of the goal, you should have a purpose for your life.

Are you an unconscious eater? Maybe food has been your ball and chain—your unconscious living—your mundane life. Release yourself of this addiction of unconscious eating and **eat to live!** To live purposefully for a common good—the Body of Christ. When this happens, your eating will not be a focal point in your life. Eating foods will be one activity of your life, and food will be a necessity—to live and not an abusive relationship with food and special treats eaten daily and unconsciously. Your eating and drinking will not be in vain, but it will give glory to God. You will begin the eating to live process—conscious eating that will help you to live out your purpose in life.

Mind over body or mind with the body

"Thy will be done in Earth as it is in Heaven."[2] Our bodies are earthly in nature, but the unseen thing—your mind and thoughts—are spiritual in nature. How do you make the two connect and work together? You do it consciously. Consciously, every member of your body knows its role and works for the common good—to be a healthy individual, both physically and spiritually. Some may call this *willpower*. Your **will** is your purpose in life, and **power** is the true execution of this will. We all have the willpower to do anything. You can fly an airplane; you can be a surgeon, teacher, scientist, a good father or mother, truck driver, janitor, nurse, pharmacist, electrician, small- or large-business owner, politician, police officer, lawyer, administrator, postal worker, accountant, or writer. Whatever your will, you have the power to do it. "I can do all things through Christ which strengthens me."[3] Allow God's <u>will</u> to be done in you and He will give you the <u>power</u> to do His will.

Also, you have the willpower to be a healthy individual! This includes being a conscious eater and not an unconscious eater.

Some observations of an unconscious eater are:
- Person is driving the car and eating french fries, doughnuts, candy bar, or hamburgers, or drinking a soda, coffee, or latté.
- People walking down the street with sodas and sipping frequently or eating their lunch on the run.
- Person cooking food and tasting and nibbling on foods throughout the cooking process and then sitting down to eat a whole meal.
- Person at work nibbling on snacks while at the computer or going to the vending machine for a snack attack.
- Person on the phone talking to relatives, friends, or co-workers while nibbling on food or drinking.
- Person entering a fast-food restaurant with a soda in their hand and ordering a combo meal that includes a second soda. Person eats combo meal, drinks two sodas, and gets a refill of soda before leaving the restaurant.
- Person eating a large meal at the table and a waitress comes around to offer a dessert, fresh-baked rolls, or sweet tea. Person accepts the offer, even though they are full.
- Person sees grease from the food through the paper bag, on their fingers, and on the plate. Grease shines on their face and lips. However, they continue to eat it.
- Person goes to the grocery store and the basket is full of snack foods, sodas, and convenience items.

- Person watching a movie or television show craves something advertised on the screen and proceeds to satisfy this false hunger with snack foods.
- Person sees some food, whether on TV, at the movies, on the kitchen table or counter, in the store's checkout line, just anywhere; therefore, the person eats it, not considering if they are hungry or need it.
- Person puts groceries in the trunk with one hand while eating a cookie from the other hand.
- Person eats their meal and nibbles on their child's uneaten food too.
- Person sips on a soda while shopping for groceries.
- Person leaves a restaurant with a to-go drink refill when they have passed the level of comfortably full.

You are what you eat. Whether you do it unconsciously or consciously, it is what it is. While willpower to some is mind over body, I question if it should be **mind and body.** They must communicate and work in unison for the common goal of eating consciously and being a healthy individual.

You can't feed your body unhealthy foods for a long period of time and say, "Why am I overweight?" Or "Why did I have a heart attack?" This condition may happen because of years of unconscious decisions. Your body will only take so much physical abuse before it will present signs and symptoms of illness or disease.

Turn this thing around!

Some examples of a conscious eater are:

- Person goes to the grocery store or local market twice a week to get fresh vegetables and fruits and prepares and eats them daily.
- Person cooks meals at least twice a week.
- Person makes a salad and enjoys all the colors, textures, and smells.
- Person goes to a restaurant that serves the right portion sizes and/ or displays calories for each menu item. In addition, the person proceeds to choose the right dish for their body's needs.

- Person drinks water throughout the day.
- Person is not preoccupied with food and waits for the next meal.
- Person passes by the vending machine and eats their prepared healthy snack or waits for the next prepared meal.
- Person is able to say **no** to foods offered that are not good for their body and knows the value of "It feels good to feel good or being comfortably full!"
- Person may become stressed but reacts by meditating, praying, or doing physical activity like walking, instead of eating unconsciously to cope with stress.

Overweight and Obesity

Overweight and Obesity are major health challenges among adults and children. Many professionals have made some strides in addressing this multi-complex health challenge through research, therapies, and practices. However, it's not enough.

Oftentimes, there is a disconnect between the various professions. A delay in disseminating useful information to those who need it is a huge problem. In addition, there are too many research projects that say "further research is needed."

Obesity/overweight is a crisis. There should be an urgency to address this chronic health challenge from the federal, state and local leaders, marketing gurus, school and community leaders, restaurants owners, food vendors, neighborhood associations, parks and recreation departments, city planning groups, police officers, and parents.

An urgent call to the parent of the child who is overweight or obese— Wake up! Wake up! The child and the child's unconscious mind have been running the show for too long. All the neighbors are shaking their heads while the child runs ravenously wild in your house/body. The child needs love, attention, and direction from the parent. The child cannot raise himself. Parents, you are the leaders. Do your job! "Train up a child in the way he should go: and when he is old, he will not depart from it."[4] The child needs discipline and he will thank you later.

All too often, we want a quick fix when it comes to overweight and dieting. Some health professionals have taken advantage of this by providing surgeries, stomach stapling, cosmetic surgery, among other treatments to trick the body and try to help the mind to get *on track*. Some of these procedures have been beneficial and life-saving for many people. However, is it the panacea of the 21st century? Can everyone afford such surgeries? Do we want bodily manipulation to be the option for chronic illnesses and diseases, which is highly preventable through behavioral modification? Many young people are suffering from major chronic diseases and illnesses such as heart disease, cancer, diabetes, asthma, blindness, nerve damage, joint problems, and other conditions. Too many young people are dying. The body is sick and needs to be healed. However, many people are focusing on the body and using it to trick the mind to do right. However, many are forgetting the *MIND!* It is the MIND that needs the help. "It's all in the Mind!" The mind is unconscious and needs an awakening—a spiritual awakening to be the parent—in control of this great body – A gift from God.

At times, you may find yourself eating something that is so good—a dessert or favorite dish—that you find yourself unable to stop eating, even when you have had enough. Also, you may experience the self-talk of "Oh this is so good!" and that self-talk overrides the feeling and awareness of "Oh, I am so stuffed—I've had enough!" This may be your struggle of doing wrong—eating too much, overindulging, "living to eat" versus wanting to do right—eating just enough—being content with "eating to live."

Your struggle is with physical self-control, but also with spiritual self-control. Oftentimes, we acknowledge the physical self-control by saying "I'm on a diet; I can't eat that" which is oftentimes temporary. As a result, you may see people who have tried diets and lost a considerable amount of weight, only to gain it back again. Why? Because it's similar to when the "check engine" light comes on in your car. You put a Band-Aid over the light, so you don't see it anymore, but the engine still needs to be fixed. Or you have a flat tire and you replace it with a spare tire but never get the regular tire fixed or replaced. Or you give a homeless person one meal for a day, but they continue to be hungry the next day. The one meal is a temporary fix. No one likes to go to the auto mechanic because of the time and possible high cost to fix the engine. *But it has to be done.* Again, to fix or replace a flat tire will require time and money. *But someone has to do it.* No one wants to take the time to teach a man how to get a job and provide for himself. *But it needs to be done.* Likewise physical self-control is a temporary fix, but the focus needs to be on spiritual self-control—

building up the mind. This will take time; it will not be easy. It may cost or cause you (the child) some discomfort momentarily, but *it has to be done—someone has to do it - It needs to be done!*

You have fallen—now get up!

If you know anyone who has fallen and bumped their head, they may have experienced temporary unconsciousness. The following are signs that indicate you are in a state of unconsciousness, especially while eating. 1. Eating just because. 2. If you have said, "Tomorrow I will start my diet" and tomorrow never comes. 3. When you have overeaten, you say, "I have fallen off the track, or I will exercise tomorrow" However, tomorrow never comes and you say "Oh well." Well, **Enough is Enough!**

You have fallen. You have gotten off the track. You have lost consciousness. You are temporarily unconscious. But Enough is Enough! Now get back up and get back on Track! Enough is Enough! There is no reason to stay unconscious or continue to sleepwalk through life. Arise and walk consciously. Be conscious of your daily decisions—have a sound mind.

Comfortably full

The body is similar to a car. Just like a car needs gas to operate, your body needs food to do daily activities. Gas is fuel for the car. Food is fuel for the body. When a car is almost on empty, the light comes on to remind the driver to get gas. Furthermore, when the car reaches empty, the car starts to drag, stall, and not perform. The driver is stuck, stranded, and stops momentarily until the car is refueled. Similarly with the body, when the body is almost on empty, hunger pangs begin and the brain receives and sends signals throughout the body as a result. When the body reaches empty, a person may start to feel weak, irritable, unable to concentrate; performance is low and the person may even faint.

Most drivers don't wait until the car is on empty before they fuel up. By the time the light comes on, the driver is looking for the next gas station to refuel. Some car owners fill up the tank, while others put in just enough for the next few errands. Whatever the situation, the driver is *aware* that the car is on empty and fuel is needed.

Unconscious eaters are not aware of the body's needs. Nonetheless, unconscious eaters do not gauge or assess the body's status to determine if it's on empty, one-quarter, one-half, three-quarters, or full. Oftentimes, unconscious eaters fuel up on foods when the body is not even hungry or when the body is full. A driver would never go to the gas station with a car already full of gas. Nor would a driver stand at the pump and allow gallons of gas to spill out of the car onto the ground when the car is full of gas. Nor will a driver put toxic substances into the car to make the car run sluggishly. However, unconscious eaters practice these daily routines by ignoring the common body cues. Carelessly, you may bypass common sense and continue to eat when the body is full and not hungry, or eat items that do not necessarily benefit the body. Thus, the body is overly full and excess calories are consumed. Also, the body is filled with foods that are low nutrients and highly dense which will make the body sluggish and not operate optimally. This is physical abuse to the body that leads to other problems down the road—some sooner rather than later.

A conscious eater has a sound mind and is aware of the body's needs. A conscious eater has a purpose in life, and food is only one component to fulfilling that purpose. Before conscious eaters sit down to eat, they already have a conscious plan of foods and drinks to be consumed and how much is needed to become comfortably full: one-quarter is needed (snack); one-half is needed (light meal); three-quarters is needed (regular meal). While they are eating, they assess the tank (stomach) and begin to listen for the same click at the gas station. The "click" sound signals that the tank is full—comfortably full. Similarly, the body feels there is enough food to supply the energy needed to accomplish the remaining activities of the day. Not too little that you feel starved, but just enough. Enough is enough. Comfortably full. A feeling of satisfaction, contentment. A body that feels light is able to accomplish more than a person that is overly full. Overly full means feeling sluggish, tired, sleepy, unable to perform, loosening of the pants, drunk with food, etc. In other words, your mind and body can be trained to be content and comfortably full. This is a process of building up your mind.

Selective Consciousness

How is it that you know the rules of the game of life, but when it comes to your body, you ignore those rules and you are unconscious in your decisions when it comes to eating. If you are late or absent from work, your paycheck will be docked—so you make it a habit to be on time. If you are driving, you know which road has the most traffic and avoid it at all costs. You program your television and computer to delete meaningless advertising. You have caller ID and screen calls of people you do not want to talk to. All of these scenarios are examples of selective conscious decisions in our daily lives. We sift through those daily activities for those things that are meaningful to us. A full paycheck, less time in traffic, commercial-free television programming and marketing-free phone calls are meaningful to many of us.

Selective conscious decisions are possible and made daily by the mind. These same decisions can be applied to our eating habits, as some are noted in chapter two. Exercise this crucial part of your body—the mind—and the other body parts will fall into place. The whole body needs to surrender! Once you have that humbling experience, your mind is ready to be reset to direct the body and provide for its needs—instead of the body directing the mind or an undisciplined child leading the parent. Your mind is capable of sifting through daily routines and making selective conscious decisions about your eating habits—to make them meaningful for your body. Why make selective conscious decisions about other parts of your life as mentioned above and then make unconscious decisions about the food you eat and your eating habits? Wake up!

Our minds are powerful when it comes to pain. The mind receives and sends messages from the body when it feels the slightest pain. We are conscious and feel pain with the smallest splinter underneath the skin; food stuck between your teeth; scrap on your elbow or knee; an eyelash in the eye; paper cut on the finger, curling iron that touches the ear; mosquito bite; bunion or callus on your feet; ingrown toe nail; and a small pimple on your back. Yet, when it comes to overeating, we tend to turn off the conscious button because our stomachs are out of sight and out of mind. So, we choose to be unconscious when we overeat and cause ourselves internal bodily discomfort and pain.

This same mind that has the power to receive and send messages about pain, especially with an eyelash in the eye is the same mind that can receive and send messages that "I am comfortably full and I need to stop eating" or "This food does not make me feel good, and I am not going to eat something that harms me" or "If I eat too much my tummy will hurt"

When something happens, like constipation, then consciousness kicks in. "I should not have eaten all those fried foods with no vegetables or water." Your conscious mind tells you, "You should have had more vegetables, fruits and water." By then, it is too late. The occurrences of constipation, heart palpitations, and other chronic illnesses and ailments have set in and become abuse to the body. When you have gout and you start to limp on one leg and soreness sets into the limbs and/or joints, your body is telling you something. If health misfortunes consistently happen over a period of time, it may cause a disease.

Consciousness is not making selective decisions when health misfortunes occur. Conscious decisions need to be selected daily for prevention today and deterrence of disease tomorrow. It should not be "I do what I want today and I will treat disease later." Feeling good, such as having regular bowel movements without constipation, is an expectation because I eat a high-fiber diet, drink water, and exercise. Healthy and sound decisions create healthy expectations. As a result, you feel good both in mind and body. Say it, "*It feels good to feel good!*"

Lust of the flesh

In the Bible, Eve allowed temptation because she was not content. She had many created things to explore in the Garden; however, the flesh was weak and so was her mind. She allowed the body (flesh) to tell the mind, "I want more; I need more." Therefore, an autopilot attitude, or an unconscious state of mind took shape. Sleepwalking caused her to get off track!

There is some truth in the popular belief of "You are powerless." However, you are powerless if you have an unconscious state of mind where the body is controlling the mind, demanding the mind/parent to be quiet while the body/child runs wild and does any- and everything—no rules, no accountability. However, there is **power** in the conscious state of mind. You are able to do all things through Christ who strengthens you![3] This is your spiritual strength—the unseen thing—spiritual muscles that need to be exercised. Your conscious mind is the unseen thing. It is also that source of natural power linked to the spiritual power or Higher Power. If you go back to the Garden/ creation and stay close to the Creator, hear His voice, meditate on Him, serve Him, do His will, do your service or talents for Him, and live with a purpose in your life, then you will be content and will not have time to fulfill the lust of the flesh or listen or yield to temptations. In essence, you will be walking in spirit and truth! You will be content in every aspect of your life, including your eating.

Consciously, your mind and body will be on one accord in eating and know when enough is enough and be satisfied and content.

Once you realize it's your spiritual being, your mind that needs to be reset, rebooted, recharged, re-energized, re-organized, refocused, restored, and revitalized, then the physical self-control will become easy and natural. The struggle to do right—eating to live and being content—versus the will to do wrong—living to eat and overindulging—will dissipate. Your will to do right will override the will to do wrong. Your strong mind—the exercised spiritual muscle, the unseen thing—will lead and the body will follow. You will establish harmony—equilibrium. Your struggle will be over. You will overcome yourself and eventually have a sound mind and body. You shall not want.[5]

Overall, you need to build up your mind, the unseen thing, and be conscious of what's going on around you. Tap into that spiritual power that is able to empower you to do things physically. Know your purpose in life. A clear purpose will guide you in this life. This clarity begins with contentment and peace with daily activities, including eating. Avoid those unconscious decisions, including poor eating habits. Allow your mind to be the leader and think consciously, but it needs to work concertedly with the body to make conscious decisions. If you are overweight, you have the willpower to overcome. Tap into the spiritual power and build up your spiritual muscles. Allow your body to experience being comfortably full and practice it daily. Train up your child/body so that God's will can be done in you.

Scripture References

1. Matthew 11:28
2. Matthew 6:10
3. Philippians 4:13
4. Proverbs 22:6
5. Psalms 23:1

CHAPTER 6
Food for the Soul
Chew on This!

Scriptures are spiritual food to build up the mind and give it the **will** and **power** it needs for a lifetime. As it was written in Chapter Two, take your time to chew physical food. Also take time to chew on God's Word and list more of your own. "Trust in the Lord with all thine heart, and lean not unto thine own understanding. In all thy ways acknowledge him and he shall direct thy paths" (Proverbs 3:5–6). "Wisdom is the principal thing, therefore get wisdom and with all thy getting get understanding" (Proverbs 4:7).

1. Genesis 1—Revelation 22
2. Joshua, Psalm, Proverbs
3. Psalm 16:3; 19:7-14; 34:8
4. Psalm119:103
5. Psalm 139:23-24
6. Proverbs 6:9; 16
7. Ecclesiastes 6:1–2, 7
8. Isaiah 55:1-11
9. Isaiah 65:17-25
10. Joel 2:12-14
11. Matthew 4:23
12. Matthew 6: 25–33
13. Matthew 7:7–11, 24-27
14. Matthew 12:33
15. Matthew 13:15—23
16. Matthew 24:14
17. Mark 12: 29–34
18. John 4:31-34
19. John 6:32–63
20. Romans 12:1-18
21. 1 Corinthians 3:16–17
22. 1 Corinthians 1:10; 6:17, 19–20;
23. 1 Corinthians 9:26-27;14:20
24. 2 Corinthians 1:3-7
25. Galatians 5:22–25
26. Ephesians 6:10-18
27. Philippians 2:1-5; 4:11–13
28. Colossians 3:10-15
29. Hebrews 6:5; 8:10;

30. Hebrews 12:1-14;13:18, 20–21
31. James 1:27; 2:8
32. 1 Peter 1:13-16; 2: 1-3; 4:1-2
33. 2 Peter 2:22
34. Revelation 2:7

See Diagram 1 in chapter 8 for more scriptures.

CHAPTER 7
Say it Again!

"Didn't I tell you to clean up this room?"

Just like a child needs repetition, your mind and body need repetition. Time is also needed to practice and practice until eating consciously is an established habit. Oftentimes, a child may hear their parents say the same message louder or softer. They may say it differently, with pictures or role playing. But the parent may have to say the same message again, over and over and over again. Sometimes a directive from a parent may be interpreted by the child differently, based on the parent's tone of voice, facial expression, and other communication formats. This purpose of this chapter is to clarify some of the previous concepts in the book. If parts of this book are vague to you, read on or have a discussion with others who have read the book. Or you may want to read on for confirmation.

Stop and Listen

So many times, parents have to remind their children of the same concepts over and over again, until they get it right. Such repetition may frustrate the parent and the child. However, a loving parent will tell the child after many attempts and many disappointments, "Keep practicing," or "Practice makes perfect," or "You will get it—don't give up!" These words of encouragement are important. One, it reminds children that they are still loved even though they may not have grasped the concepts and not feel that they have disappointed their parent or themselves. Also, the power or authority remains with the parent. The parent is in charge, not the child. Sometimes, it's hard as parents to see your efforts because your child is not making progress fast enough or none at all. Oftentimes, parents feel overwhelmed with the process and either they want to step in and help the child or revert back to the child running the show, doing childish things. It is bittersweet. Parents know that if they sit back and coach the child from the sidelines, the child will become strong through his trials and failures. It will make them better children. Often, children will remember those encouraging words when they become adults, experiencing similar trials and tribulations but on another level. On the other side, children may become overwhelmed with their need to succeed, and experience disappointments. As a result, they continually beg for their parents' help or they do not communicate at all. So the child never completes the growing process or experiences the next level of maturation. The parent continues to provide for the child and as a result, the parent relinquishes authority and the child has the power. So instead of the child facing various variable, i.e., life challenges and disappointments, the child wants to be a child and play, play, play with no rules, no discipline, just feel good all the time with no responsibilities or decisions—The parent and child slip into a mode of unconsciousness. Unconscious of the situation, unconscious of making the right decisions, unconscious of life—darkness, sleepwalking, doing things with no strings attached—automatic life – a mindless existence. Therefore, somethng is "on," but it is not the parent. It is the lust of the flesh! Lust. The child says, "I want, I need, I must have," etc. and the child gets it while the parent is asleep! The parent is "off" the job of discipline, order, rules, guidance—all out of love. Love for self. Love for the child, love for the body, vessel, temple, a Godly gift given to you.

Who has to stop and listen? The parent has to tune in to the true needs of the body, not the presumptuous lust of the flesh but the true hunger and thirst for God. God's spirit will lead and guide you into all truth and righteousness. The child has to stop and listen to the parent's guidance. When the parent says the stove is hot, it is dangerous. The child must believe the parent is telling him right things, good things to keep him out of harm's way. Stop and listen. The child must realize he does not have the understanding of the parent yet. So the parent's guidance is crucial to the child's survival. A child can't live without it. Once order is established, including a set protocol, then the body and soul are sound and they walk in unison together. They ultimately hear God's voice and instruction. The mind and body are now a part of God's creation. This body knows its Creator and understands His plan—to love God with all your mind, body, and soul and to love your neighbor as yourself.

A reunion is created. A spiritual reunion is formed like the prodigal son who left and found his way back to his father. A reunion like the one lost sheep of the one hundred that was then found; even the angels rejoiced. It is a reunion, because now you look into the perfect law of liberty—a mirror image of God. A freedom to know good has conquered evil. Now you walk freely before God. You walk in the Spirit and perfect before Him.[1-2] You walk holy because He is holy.[3-4] Your spiritual reunion becomes a joy because you are made in the very image of God[5], and the Kingdom of God is inside of *you!* [6]

We are members of the body of Christ. Everyone has a goal or purpose in order for the body to function. The eye cannot boast without the finger.

The finger cannot boast without the arm, etc. We all need one another to glorify the body of Christ![7-9] Therefore, the kingdom of heaven is within us.[7,10] We are the temples.[11] We must present our bodies a living sacrifice unto God. We are the sanctuaries that give sacrifices of praise and song.[12-13] People need to see God's light within us. His light, not darkness. We are children of the light.[14] "For ye were sometimes in darkness, but now are ye light in the Lord: walk as children of the light. For the fruit of the Spirit is in all goodness and righteousness and truth; Proving what is acceptable unto the Lord. And have no fellowship with the unfruitful works of darkness, but rather reprove them."[15]

What is your purpose when food is not your focal point? When you are at ground zero, fasting, when you have a clear mind, what is your purpose in the body of Christ? What light do people see inside of you? What savor/salt do you have? What sacrifices do you have for the Lord? For it is better to obey than to sacrifice. Are you obeying? Are you listening to God's words, voice, and laws? Are you giving sacrifices of joy and praise? What talent or gift has He given you? Are you using your gift? How are you pleasing God? What is your reasonable service?

Out of sight, out of mind - A

Why is it that we think we are in control when we are not? Many of us have health problems such as constipation, yet we continue to eat a diet of processed foods and no fiber or water. We have high blood pressure, yet we continue to eat salty and processed foods. We are overweight and may have diabetes, yet we continue to eat cookies, candies, sodas, and large servings of food. We have yeast infections, yet we eat sweetened products; tooth decay, yet we continue to eat sticky foods and sweetened foods and beverages. We have brittle bones, yet we continue to consume a diet with little or no calcium. We get heartburn, yet we continue to eat large meals, spicy foods, or late at night. Despite gout, we continue to consume a rich diet of meats and sweetened products, and the list goes on. Most of all, we do not drink enough water or get enough exercise.

The evidence is in the sales of hemorrhoid medicines and stool softeners to relieve constipation, acid reflux medication for heartburn, blood pressure medicine and yeast infection medicine, and the list goes on. We are addicted to pain and agony, and use whatever medicines and resources that are available to rid us of the pain. (If you look at commercials and advertisements for some of these products, you will see the truth in the addiction to pain and agony: eat all you want and feel bad, and we have the product to help you feel better.)

Ultimately, the child messes up the house through unconscious eating, and the parent pays good money to clean it up. The house (body) gets temporary fixes to the problems. However, the parent has got to say *enough is enough! I don't want to keep cleaning and fixing up the house. The plumbing is bad, the electrical wires are bad, sewage is backed up, and pests are in the house* (flies, rodents, and roaches). Just because you don't see it does not mean it's not happening or occurring in your body. Enough is enough. We want a clean and functioning house/body, not one full of potential hazards such as health problems that lead to chronic diseases.

The inside of your body is out of sight, so it's out of mind. The inside of your body comes to mind mostly when illness or disease sets in, and then reversing the condition and lifestyle becomes a Herculean effort to correct. For instance, your heart becomes precious to you when you need heart surgery; your kidneys become precious to you when you need dialysis; your colon becomes precious to you when you need a colostomy; your blood and blood vessels in your eyes, hands and feet are precious to you when you have uncontrolled diabetes, etc. Even though your inner body parts are out of sight, do not put them out of your mind. They need the mind to take care of them.

Put a mental mirror up to the inside of your body. What do you see? Better yet, go to the clinic and get health screenings on cholesterol, LDL, HDL, TG, blood pressure, blood sugar, BMI, kidney tests, waist circumference, bone density, etc. What is your family history? What is your reflection? What do you see in your mental mirror of yourself on the inside? Do you like what you see in that mirror? If not, do something. Turn this thing around and do something! Whether it's for prevention or treatment, your inside body needs just as much attention and love as the outer body and appearance. Do something! Keep that mental reflection/picture of the inside body in your mind so you can start to make conscious decisions about your eating habits. If you do not, it will be out of sight and out of mind. The child will be in control and unconscious decisions will be made.

Out of sight, out of mind – B

When you go to the grocery store, corner store, or gas station to shop, what are you shopping for? What type of foods, drinks, and snacks are in your basket, brown bag, or hand? Who made the purchase decision to buy those items? Was it the parent or was it the child? If your purchases are mostly snacks foods or drinks with very few nutrients or the purchase decision was bought because of emotions and not based on your body's need for energy, then your unconscious drive for poor eating habits is great and so are the temptations. Once these foods are purchased and enter your possession, the mind has to constantly battle over the consumption of when? and how much? This battle or struggle will be a constant nag in the mind if low nutrient/high dense foods are in sight and readily available in the car; at the desk or computer; and in the kitchen cabinets, refrigerator or freezer. If these foods are out of sight, then they are out of mind. Temptations will decline. Over time your mind will be strengthen as you practice the behavior of purchasing foods or drinks that are meaningful for your body. This behavior will become a natural habit with time and patience. Eventually, your foggy thoughts and mundane actions will decrease while your clarity will increase and mind muscles strengthened. You will have less time to spend on the struggles of food and more time to spend on other areas of your life. Self love becomes evident and your purpose in life becomes alive and fruitful to you, others, and your Creator.

My Struggles

My struggles are not unique. Like most people, I have tasted food while preparing it for my family, not realizing that I was already comfortably full by the time I sat down to eat with them. I have eaten food or had a soft drink to relieve stress. I have gone to an all-you-can-eat restaurant. I had every intention of eating a salad but was tantalized by the many choices and I ignored the warnings from my mind (parent) that I was more than comfortably full. I have given in to the wants of the child, conned into the belief that in order to get my money's worth, I had to eat desserts that I don't normally eat or care to bake. Some days I have found myself too tired to cook, and gone through the drive-thru of a fast-food restaurant to get something quick and easy, not questioning the calories or its nutritional value to the body. I enjoy eating cold foods like ice cream, yogurt, and smoothies, but am unconscious of how much I am eating or drinking because it is my pleasurable eating period. I like vegetarian foods, especially foods that include a lot of spices, but because it is vegetarian food and noted as being healthy, my body has tricked my mind into believing that I can have more of it. Suffice it to say, I have been a prisoner in my own home—my body; a prisoner of the child who makes decisions for the parent. Until one day, I realized that the parent was back from vacation. The parent was ready with love to take on the responsibilities to lead and guide the body (child) in the right direction. In other words, the mind is ready to make sound decisions for the body.

My struggles were in both my mind and body. In my mind, I was weak and unconscious of my eating habits. I didn't want to think about organizing one more part of my life. I was organized at work and somewhat at home, and it became overwhelming just being a woman in life. So I would rather not organize my eating habits and set parameters of what I eat—just let my hair down and not think about a food plan for my body. It was not abnormal for me to eat whatever, whenever, and as much as I wanted to eat. However, it was abnormal because I did it too often and I often felt guilty afterward. Also, I felt like a hypocrite.

I should have an eating plan, but I wish someone could do it for me. It's so hard to be a woman, with all the demands of life. I know I have a family history of medical problems and I have to eat right to prevent some of the same chronic illnesses and diseases from happening to me. Somehow, there is a disconnect between my mind and body. I want to be whole; I want my mind and body to be strong and to have the courage to change the things I can change. I can plan and prepare and eat healthy meals. I can exercise more; I can do more for myself. I have the privilege to care for me, then I will not be a burden to myself, others or society. I will become a source of love and give God the praise, honor and glory and be able to help someone else. My struggles will be over because I press toward the mark – I will overcome.

Are you sick?

When people have a cold or the flu, they use all types of natural and traditional remedies to get well again. Many use healthy foods to build up the body's immune system to get well. Oftentimes, a good night's rest is good for the body to improve its immune system. The body is receptive to this care, and it craves this attention—attention from the mind, from others caring for you! Your body is recuperating from the overwhelming demands of taking care of everyone's needs and desires and saying to you, "Hey, I need you to take care of me!"

So what? You do not have a cold or flu, but are you sick? You may be sick and don't even know it. Sometimes the mind is receiving signals of pain and discomfort – illnesses, but the body overrides these signals. If you are sick with illnesses, as discussed before in this book, do something about it. Your body may be craving for attention. Don't wait until the pain or discomfort is so unbearable that you have to go to the doctor or hospital before you wake up! Wake up now—on this side — prevention and not treatment!

While you don't have symptoms of a cold or flu, you may have symptoms of chronic diseases. Even if you do not have any symptoms, your body needs attention: to be fed healthy things to stay healthy. Just as a car needs the oil changed every three thousand miles or three months, your body needs maintenance. Just as a house may have termite damage but the homeowner does not know it, you may have internal damage, i.e., symptoms of chronic diseases that you do not know about. This body needs maintenance, just like a car. You need regular checkups (health inspections), just like a house inspection detect pest and structural damage that are not easily seen. You are an investment—God's investment. Would you conduct reckless behaviors with an investment? No! It's the same scenario when you eat.

You would not feed yourself with snack foods on a regular basis when you are sick with a cold or flu. During this illness, every food or drink you consume is with a purpose—to get well. Now, turn it around! Every food and drink you consume when you are not sick should be for a purpose—to stay well—maintain good health—energy to live! Wake up! Ask yourself if you are sick. Do you need maintenance? Do you need a health inspection?

Summary

First the parent realized that this body was temporary and a gift from God. This gift is special, and great care goes into accepting this gift. Next, the parent had to erase or disconnect the images of things that do not benefit the body—like memories of daily pleasurable eating and set rules to reboot, re-organize, rebuild the mind and body. Developing a spiritual connection is necessary by establishing ground zero through fasting and praying. This establishes a purpose in life of love: love for self, love for God, and love for one's neighbor. When this purpose of life is established, it conjures a clearer walk in the Spirit unobstructed from fulfilling the lust of the flesh. This is achieved by beginning a spiritual walk in the scriptures—eating God's Word daily. Also, it can be a physical walk in nature to see God's gifts to you: trees, flowers, insects, sky, clouds, sun, moon, stars, grass, rivers, lakes, streams, mountains, and even the simple air that we breathe (but do not see). All of these things were created just for you. No one wants to be poor in anything, but when you are poor and realize that you can do something about it, you take advantage of it. God's Word was there all the time. Consuming God's Word—spiritual food for the soul—is your escape from the lust of the flesh and a development of a stronger spiritual connection. Your hunger and thirst become stronger for spiritual things such as righteousness. You develop stronger muscles in the spiritual body when you consume this spiritual bread and water. Finally, you develop a pure heart like a child. You are innocent and seek guidance not only from the conscious mind but also from the Spiritual being that created you.

These spiritual *acknowledgments* can be a foundation to which you can start to live consciously. Consciously you become aware of the *truths* that have been with you all along. For instance, "don't eat too much or your belly will hurt." Parents know this and try to help the child to avoid such pain and agony. God, the Higher Power, can lead and direct you in all things, including eating. Tapping into that source of power enables you to have the **will** and **power** to do anything, including being healthy, and a desire to prevent pain and agony of chronic disease.

In essence, It is all about You! Take a look on the inside. What is your reflection? If you were given a mirror, what would the mirror tell you about yourself on the inside, both spiritually and physically? Just as you would look in the mirror before you leave the house and correct your hair, tie, dress, collar, makeup, etc., if you see flaws in the mental mirror of your spiritual and physical (inner and outer) body, then change your thought process, redirect your thoughts, and become more aware of your eating habits, and do things that demonstrate a true reflection of who you want to be: conscious eater, healthy individual, living with a purpose in this life. You are what you eat.

To stay on this path, it is important to continue to meditate on God's word—this is your ultimate source of food for the soul. "Man shall not live by bread alone, but by every WORD that proceedeth out of the mouth of God."[16]

"Beloved, I wish above all things that thou
mayest prosper and be in health,
even as thy soul prospereth." [17]

Scripture References

1. Romans 8:4
2. Matthew 5:48
3. Leviticus 11:44
4. 1 Peter 1:16
5. Genesis 1:26-27
6. Luke 17:21
7. Romans 12:4-21
8. 1 Corinthians 6:19-20
9. Colossians 3:13–17
10. Mark 12:29-34
11. 1 Corinthians 3:16–17
12. Romans 12:1
13. Hebrews 13:15-16
14. John 12:35–36
15. Ephesians 5:8–20
16. Matthew 4:4
17. 3 John 1:2

Say It Again Statements

"It's all in my Mind!"

"Just push away"

"Who is the parent?"

"Child, sit down to eat, chew your food, eat your vegetables and fruits today, don't eat late at night, enough is enough....."

"Do what I say!"

"Little child, little child. Listen to me"

"I am in control!"

"Enough is Enough"

"I can do this!"

"Help Me Lord!"

"Comfort Me, Oh Lord when I cry!"

"Yes, Jesus Love Me!"

"I surrender"

"I need help!"

"Go to bed!"

"Take a deep breath."

"Close up the refrigerator"

"If it's not in the house then you don't have to worry about it."

"I need fruits and vegetables in the house"

"Drink some water"

"It's Me, Oh Lord, standing in the need of prayer!"

"His mercy endureth forever"

"I got work to do!" Time with family and friends, Time for Charity, Chores around the house, Office work, etc.

"My purpose in life is _____"

"I am about my Father's business"

"I've got to turn this thing around"

"When I want to do wrong, Help me to do right!"

"Not my will Lord, but your will!"

"It's all about Me!"

"It's all about You - Jesus!"

CHAPTER 8
Picture it Again!

Pictures tell the whole story

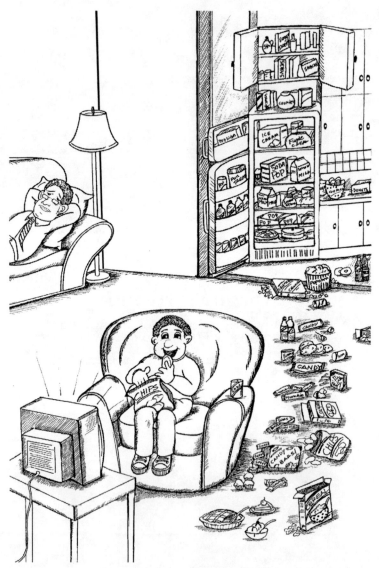

The parent is unconscious while the child is in control or out of control. Wake up! Turn this thing around!

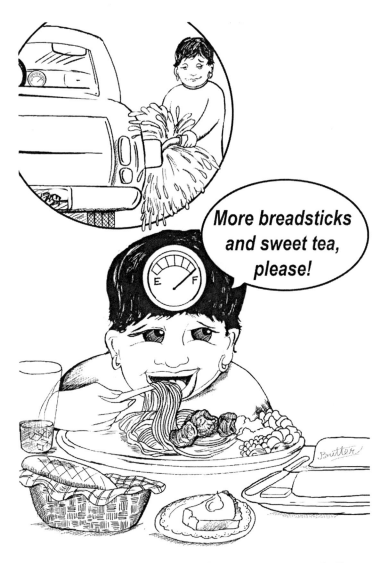

"Would you pump gas into a car that is on **FULL** and allow it to spill out? So, why allow your body to eat when it is **FULL**? This is unconscious behavior. Wake up! Turn this thing around!

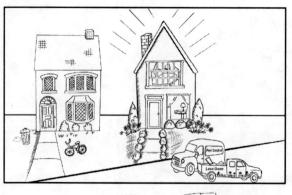

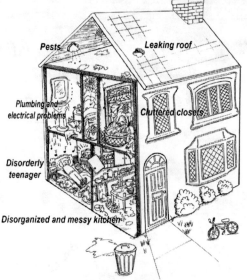

"The first house gives the outer appearance of being maintained but on the inside of the house there are serious concerns that have gone unnoticed. The other house gets regular attention and is well maintained and problems are prevented before they get out of control. What is going on in your house—BODY?"

Scripture References
Matthew 23:25-28, 38
Hebrew 3:4-6
1 Peter 2:4-9; 3:1-4

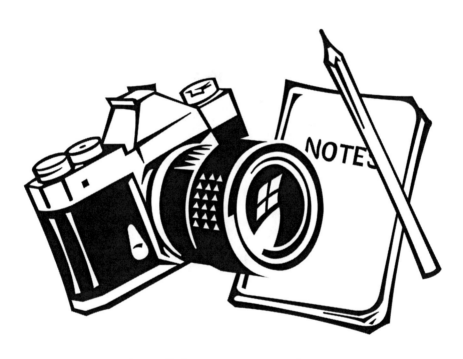

What will the camera capture about you?
A picture will tell the story.

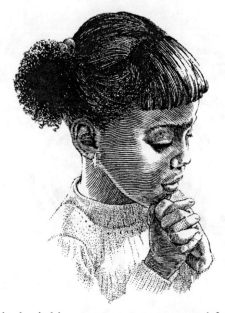

"Suffer the little children to come unto me, and forbid them not: for of such is the kingdom of God." Mark 10:14

You are
What you Eat

SIT DOWN TO EAT

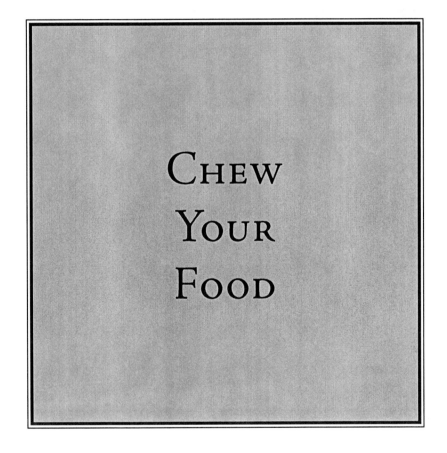

CHEW
YOUR
FOOD

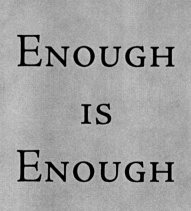

ENOUGH
IS
ENOUGH

Conscious, Health and Spiritual Map
Where am I?

Conscious, Health and Spiritual Map

Lifetime ⟶ | The Transformation – Born Again! | **Eternal Life**

Spiritual

Lifetime – FEEL BAD!	Lifetime – FEEL GOOD!	Eternal Life
Confusion	Peace	Peace – which passeth all understanding
Unlawful	Law	No laws
Sacrifices	Obedience	Sacrifices of Praise
Curses	Blessings	Blessing from God – Salvation
Dry Bones	Earthly Body	Heavenly Body
No Flavor	Salt of the Earth	Inherit the Kingdom
Darkness	Light	Children of the Light
Dead Tree	Good Seed / Ground	Fruitful Tree
Goat	Sheep	Good and Faithful Servant
Hearer – Glass	Doer – Mirror	Created in God's Image
Rebellious Child	Obedient Child	Children of God – God Family
High Level of Pain and Agony	High Level of Healthy Habits	

Health

FEEL BAD!	FEEL GOOD!
Low Level of Healthy Habits	Low Level of Pain and Agony

TURN THIS THING AROUND! – WAKE UP!

THE STRUGGLE

Consciousness

FEEL BAD!	FEEL GOOD!
Child	Man
Unconscious	Conscious
Unaware	Self Awareness
Autopilot – Cruise Control	Conscious Behavior
Addictive Behavior	Productive Behavior
"I want I want!"	"Enough is Enough"
No Purpose in Life	Purpose in Life

Diagram 1 Conscious, Health and Spiritual Map. Some people have read a map in the mall, amusement park or college campus. Usually, it reads "You are Here" with a red mark. Review the Conscious, Health and Spiritual Map. Ask yourself, "Where am I?" and "Where do I want to be?"

Map Reference

Confusion/Peace
- Romans 2:8-10
- Romans 8:4-6
- 1 Corinthians 14:33
- Philippians 4:7
- 2 Thessalonians 3:11-12
- James 3:16-18

Unlawful/Law/No Laws
- Deuteronomy 4:1,2, 5-8
- Deuteronomy 6:1-3, 24-25
- Joshua 1:7
- Jeremiah 31:33
- Jeremiah 44:10, 23
- Matthew 5:17
- Romans 7:12
- Galatians 5:22-23

Sacrifice/Obedience/Praise
- 1 Samuel 15:22
- Isaiah 1:11-18
- Jeremiah 7:22-23
- Micah 6:6-8
- 1 Corinthians 9:27

Curses/Blessings
- Deuteronomy 28:1-68
- Matthew 25: 31-40

Dry Bones/Earthly Body/Heavenly Body
- Ezekiel 37:1-14
- 1 Corinthians 15:44-49

No Flavor/Salt of the Earth/Inherit the Kingdom
- Matthew 5:13
- Matthew 5:6

- Matthew 25:34

Darkness/Light/Children of the Light
- Matthew 5:14-16
- John 12:35-36
- Ephesians 6:11-12

Stony Ground-Dead Tree/Good Ground-Seed/Fruit Tree
- Psalm 1:1-3
- Jeremiah 17:7-8
- Matthew 7:17-20
- Matthew 12:33
- Matthew 13:3-9; 18-30; 37-38
- Matthew 21:18-19
- Luke 13:6-9
- Luke 17:21
- Luke 20:34-36
- 1 Corinthians 15:35-38
- Galatians 5:22
- 1 Peter 2:9

Goat /Sheep/Good and Faithful servant
- Matthew 25:21, 23, 31-40

Hearer/Doer/Created in His image
- Genesis 1:26
- 1 Corinthians 15:47-50
- James 1:22-25

Rebellious Child/Obedient Child/Children of God
- Isaiah 30:1-3; 8-9
- Jeremiah 7:23
- Ezekiel 2:8
- Matthew 12:49-50; 18:1-5
- 1 Peter 1:14-16
- Revelation 21:7

The Struggle/Wake Up!/Turn This Thing Around!
- 2 Chronicles 7:14
- Proverbs 1:23; 26:11
- Jeremiah 3:14; 25:5; 26:3
- Ezekiel 18:31-32
- Ezekiel 33:11
- Joel 2:12-14
- Romans 7:7-25; 13:11
- 2 Peter 2:22

Transformation/Born Again!
- John 3:3-8
- 1 Corinthians 15:47-58

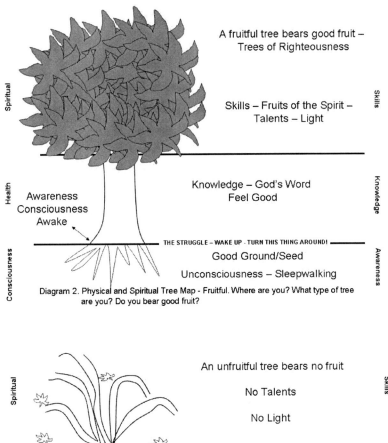

A fruitful tree bears good fruit –
Trees of Righteousness

Skills – Fruits of the Spirit –
Talents – Light

Spiritual

Skills

Health

Knowledge

Knowledge – God's Word
Feel Good

Awareness
Consciousness
Awake

Consciousness

Awareness

THE STRUGGLE – WAKE UP - TURN THIS THING AROUND!

Good Ground/Seed

Unconsciousness – Sleepwalking

Diagram 2. Physical and Spiritual Tree Map - Fruitful. Where are you? What type of tree are you? Do you bear good fruit?

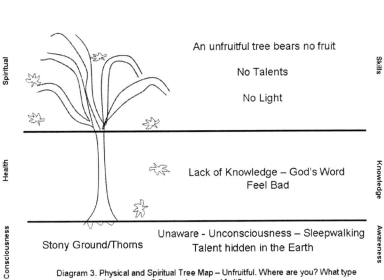

An unfruitful tree bears no fruit

No Talents

No Light

Spiritual

Skills

Health

Knowledge

Lack of Knowledge – God's Word
Feel Bad

Consciousness

Awareness

Unaware - Unconsciousness – Sleepwalking

Stony Ground/Thorns

Talent hidden in the Earth

Diagram 3. Physical and Spiritual Tree Map – Unfruitful. Where are you? What type of tree are you? Do you bear good fruit?

Scripture References

Genesis 1:26-29
Psalm 1:1-3
Proverbs 11:30
Song of Solomon 4:12-16
Matthew 7:17-20
Matthew 9:37-38
Matthew 12:33
Matthew 13:18-23; 31-32
Matthew 25:14-30
Mark 4:14-20; 26-32
Mark 8:22-25
John 15:1-15
Galatians 5:22-24
James 3:17-18
2 Peter 1:1-8
Jude 1:2
Revelation 2:7
Revelation 22:1-2

CHAPTER 9
It's All about Me!

Turn this thing around!

It's all about me!
It's all about me!
It's ALL about me!

God knew me before my father and mother knew me.
He created me in my mother's womb.[0]
God knew me before my husband knew me.
God knew me before I had my two sons!

It's ALL about me!

God told me, not Moses,
To love Him with all my heart, all my soul, and all my mind.
He told me to love my neighbor as myself.[1]
You see, when I am at work and my supervisor or
co-workers are giving me grief,
or when I am on I-285 and that person cuts me off,
makes me want to H-O-L-L-A but instead

It's ALL about me!

It's about me having praise in my heart during my trials and
tribulations.[2]
It's about me having a song on my mind,
and a smile to supervisor or co-workers on the job.
It's about me waving hello or blowing a kiss to the
person who cuts me off.

It's ALL about me!

You see
It's about me submitting to my husband[3] so he may see Christ in me!
It's about me when my children don't want to listen.
See, God told me to train up my children
in the way that they should go
So when they are old, they will not depart from it.[4]

It's ALL about me!

God told me to fear Him, and this is the beginning of knowledge.[5]
He told me to pray and fast.[6]
He told me to love Him with all my heart,
all my soul, and all my mind.[1]
He told me to love my neighbor as myself.[1]
He told me that whatever I eat or drink or whatever I do,
Do it to the glory of God![7]
He told me to walk in the Spirit and not fulfil the lust of the flesh.[8]
He told me He was the Bread of Life—the words that He speaks,
they are spirit and they are life.[9]
He told me that man shall not live by bread alone, but by every word
that proceedeth out of His mouth.[10]
He told me that he provides water that
springs up into everlasting life.[11]
He told me to hunger and thirst after righteousness and
I shall be filled.[12]
He told me to have a pure heart[13]
To seek His kingdom and His righteousness and all these things shall
be added unto me.[14]

It's ALL about me!

You see, when I am stressed out at work,
When my husband won't do right,
When my children won't listen,
When things go wrong,
When things go right,
It's all about me!

It is me who has to make the right decisions,
It is me who has to make the right decisions,
Create in me a clean heart.[15]
So I rejoice not in iniquity but rejoice in the truth,
Beareth all things, believeth all things, hopeth all things,
Endureth all things[16]

When I was a child, I spake as a child I understood as a child,
I thought as a child; but when I became a WOMAN [MAN],
I put away childish things.[17]

It is me who has to be conscious and eat the right things.
It is me buying good foods from the grocery store.
It is me preparing healthy foods for me and my family.
It is me who sits down to the table and thanks the Good Lord.
It is me who eats my vegetables and fruits.
It is me who drinks clean water.
It is me who chews my foods properly.
It is me who eats or drinks calcium-rich foods and drinks.
It is me who drinks juice as a treat.
It is me who said enough is enough.

It's about me praying to God; praying with my partner;
Having Friends who have God's Light in them;
Participating in a support group;
Sharing my food with others; being physically active;
And meditating on good things!

It's all about me!
It's ALL about me!

You see, I've got to turn this thing around.
I've got to turn it around
I've got to turn it around
For the good that I would—I do not:
but the evil which I would not, I do.
When I want to do right, I find that evil is present with me.[18]

Ah!!! There is my struggle.
Ahh!! There is my struggle.

Surely you're turning of things upside down
shall be esteemed as the potter's clay:
For shall the work say of him that made it, He made me not? Or shall
the thing framed say to him that framed it,
He had no understanding.[19]
The Spirit is willing but the flesh is weak.[20]

Wake up!
Wake up!
Wake up!
Turn this thing around.
Turn this thing around.

Yes, we know that all things work together
for good to them that love God,
to them who are called according to His purpose.
Who shall separate us from the love of Christ?
Shall tribulation, or distress, or persecution,
or famine, nakedness, or peril, or sword?
For I am persuaded that neither death nor life nor angels
nor principalities nor powers
nor things present nor things to come nor height nor depth
nor any other creature shall be able to separate us
from the love of God, which is in Christ Jesus our Lord![21]

Wake up!
Wake up!
Wake up!
Turn this thing around.
Turn this thing around.

You are the Cornerstone.[22]
If I can just lay one stone,
If I can just lay one stone,[23]

93

You see if I turn this thing around and
Go around *right* the first time
Once ENOUGH!

It is me who wants to serve God with all my heart,
all my soul, all my mind, and all of my strength
It is me who wants to love my neighbor as myself.[24]

Yes, it's me! It's me, Oh Lord.
Standing in the need of prayer
Yes, it's me! It's me, Oh Lord.
Standing in the need of prayer.
It's not my father or my mother
But it's me, Oh Lord,
Standing in the need of prayer.
It's not my brother or my sister
But it's me, Oh Lord,
Standing in the need of prayer.

It's all about me!

Yes, Jesus loves ME
Yes, Jesus loves ME
Yes, Jesus loves ME
For the Bible tells ME so!

See y'all not hearing me. I got to turn this thing around.

Finally, brethren,
whatsoever things are true, whatsoever things are honest,
whatsoever things are just, whatsoever things are pure,
whatsoever things are lovely, whatsoever things are of good report;
if there be any virtue,
and if there be any praise *Think* on these things.[25]

It's ALL about me.

You see, it's not about my father or my mother,
It's not about my brothers or my sisters,
It's not about my husband or my sons,
It's not about my supervisor or my co-workers,
It's not about the stranger who wants to cut me off.
It's all about me!

Help me, Lord
Help me, Lord
When I want to do wrong,
Help me to do Right
When I want to do wrong,
Help me to do Right
'Cause it's about me, oh Lord.

I say it again:
When I want to do right,
Evil is present with me.
When I want to do right,
Evil is present with me.
My members war against each other[26]
It's all in the mind!
I must be transformed by the renewing of
My MIND![27]

People need to see You, oh Lord, inside of me!
They need to see your light inside of me.
Help me to be one of the children of the light.[28]
You said you would be a lamp unto my feet
And a light unto my pathway.[29]
Let my delight be in you.[30]

Help me, oh Lord!
'Cause its all about me
Serving you
All my members from my head to my toes
serving you.

Help me so I can give you all the
Glory, honor, and praise.

You see, when the Lord comes again,
I want Him to look at ME.
Look at me!
Even me
Even me
Even me, oh Lord!
And say to ME

You fought a good fight![31]
You endured until the end![32]
You overcame![33]
Well done, my good and faithful servant![34]

It's ALL about YOU![35]

Scripture References

Psalm 51:1-5
1. Matthew 22:37, 39
2. Matthew 5:11-12; Romans 5:3-5; 1 Peter 3:13-17
3. Ephesians 5:22
4. Proverbs 22:6
5. Proverbs 1:7
6. Mark 9:29
7. 1 Corinthians 10:31
8. Galatians 5:16
9. John 6:48, 63
10. Deuteronomy 8:3; Luke 4:4
11. John 4:14
12. Matthew 5:6
13. Matthew 5:8
14. Luke 12:31
15. Psalms 51:10
16. 1 Corinthians 13:6-7
17. 1 Corinthians 13:11
18. Romans 7:19–21
19. Isaiah 29:16
20. Matthew 26:41
21. Romans 8:28, 35, 38–39
22. Ephesians 2:20–22
23. 1 Peter 2:5
24. Mark 12:29-34
25. Philippians 4:8
26. Romans 7:23; James 4:1-8
27. Romans 12:2
28. Matthew 5:9; John 12:36
29. Psalms 119:105
30. Romans 7:22
31. 1 Timothy 6:12
32. Matthew 24:13
33. Revelation 2:7, 11, 17, 26; 3:5, 12, 21
34. Matthew 25:23
35. Colossians 3:1-24

PART 3:
SKILLS
GROW A GARDEN

USES OF THIS BOOK

There are various uses for this book. This book may be used:

1. To increase your awareness of conscious eating. Nothing more and nothing less: an increase of awareness.

2. To help you understand the struggles between the parent and child, mind and body, and spiritual and physical.

3. To redirect your ways to conscious eating habits. You may start by writing down the struggles of your current eating habits and trying to set a goal or goals of what type of eating habits you envision and want to establish after you read this book (track record).

4. As a workbook, by cutting out the acknowledgments and truths in the back of the book. A person may want to write down other acknowledgments and truths that are personal to him or her. Others may want to write down their conscious and unconscious decisions about their daily eating habits. Establish a track record of an eating plan tailored for you. Or share your thoughts, struggles, and victories in a group setting.

5. To assist the reader in finding a new purpose in life rather than a primary focus on unconscious eating.

6. To review and obtain more scriptures—"soul food"—and gain strength to fight spiritual and physical struggles.

7. To help people better understand physical and spiritual self-control by learning to build up the mind.

8. To help people better understand various concepts through illustrations.

9. To acknowledge the Mind, Body and Spirit in addressing overweight and obesity which is a multi-complex health challenge.

10. To renew or find a new spiritual foundation of freedom, hope, faith, praise, song, and have a better understanding of the magnificent gift that was given to the you—your **mind** and **body.**

RESOURCES

NOW, CAN YOU HEAR ME?

While this book does not promote any diet plan or nutrition therapy, there are several good resources to assist the reader if one desires such a plan, therapy, or support. The purpose of this book was to take a step back from all the current issues surrounding diet, eating, overweight, obesity, weight-loss strategies, etc., and deal solely with the individual's state of mind. Become conscious of your eating habits and understand the concepts of eating consciously. After the concepts are received and understood, it is hoped that the reader can seek and accept good resources readily available, that you may be able to apply to your life. After all, it's all about YOU! This is where the rubber meets the road. Instead of a disconnect as discussed earlier, the author hopes for a connection between the reader and the various resources readily available to everyone to put into action.

Also, many people who have experienced dieting or weight loss and have gained it back may say, "I fell off the wagon" or "I fell off the track." Well, my question to you is what is your wagon? What is your track? Many people know that they have fallen off the track, but may not have a track or are lost and can't find the track. If you do not have a track to follow, you are bound to be unconscious and sleepwalking and have a track record of failure.

Many people have unique eating habits, cultural food practices, and some dietary restrictions. So I encourage you to discover and embrace your TRACK-EATING PLAN that is tailored to you. You need a plan that you can incorporate daily in your lifestyle. Write it down, make a mental note of it and speak it out loud. Once you have established a plan that works for you, then with love, you can guide your body to better eating habits—eating consciously. Also, you will consciously know when you have fallen off the *wagon* or *track* and you will have a track record that will guide you back to the lifestyle that you desire to live.

Now, go and turn this thing around!

SOME RESOURCES

AMERICA ON THE MOVE
www.americaonthemove.org

BEST OF LIFE
www.thebestlife.com

FIRST PLACE 4 HEALTH
www.firstplace.org

OVEREATERS ANONYMOUS
www.oa.org

REGISTERED DIETITIANS (RD)
www.eatright.org

TOPS
www.tops.org

U.S. OBESITY TRENDS 1985–2008
POWERPOINT SLIDE PRESENTATION
www.cdc.gov/obesity/data/trends.html

USDA FOOD GUIDE PYRAMID
www.mypyramid.gov

WEIGHT WATCHERS
www.weightwatchers.com

YMCA
www.ymca.net

Resources were accessed October 24, 2009.

Appendix A

Acknowledgments

Acknowledgment 1
The fear of the Lord is the beginning of knowledge: but fools despise wisdom and instruction.
Proverbs 1:7

Acknowledgment 2
This kind can come forth by nothing, but by prayer and fasting.
Mark 9:29

Acknowledgment 3
Whether therefore ye eat, or drink, or whatsoever ye do,
do all to the glory of God.
1 Corinthians 10:31

Acknowledgment 4
Thou shalt love the Lord thy God with all thy heart, and with all thy soul, and with all thy mind ... Thou shalt love thy neighbor as thyself.
Matthew 22:37–40

Acknowledgment 5
Walk in the Spirit, and ye shall not fulfill the lust of the flesh.
Galatians 5:16

Acknowledgment 6
Blessed are the poor in Spirit for theirs is the kingdom of heaven.
Matthew 5:3

Acknowledgment 7
Blessed are they which do hunger and thirst after righteousness:
for they shall be filled.
Matthew 5:6

Acknowledgment 8
Blessed are the pure in heart: for they shall see God.
Matthew 5:8

Appendix B

Truths

Truth 1
You are what you eat.

Truth 2
Eat all of your vegetables and fruits.

Truth 3
Don't eat too much or your tummy will hurt!

Truth 4
Eat to live and not live to eat.

Truth 5
Sit down to eat.

Truth 6
Chew your food.

Truth 7
Your skin looks terrible; stop drinking all that soda. Drink water!

Truth 8
Don't eat late at night.

Truth 9
Drink your milk!

Truth 10
Eat your food before you drink your juice.

**Truth 11
Enough is Enough.**

**Truth 12
Bonus
Go outside and PLAY!**

Appendix C

Fasting

Fasting should not be used as a form of weight loss. The fasting process is a personal experience and a spiritual and physical connection between you, your body, and God. It will help you to develop a closer relationship with God and build up the conscious mind. Below are a few suggestions.

1. Consult with your medical doctor/healthcare provider about your desire to fast, especially if you have any medical conditions, i.e., cancer, diabetes, eating disorders, etc. Talk to them specifically about fasting, the reason why you want to fast, and the plan to fast.

2. If approved by your healthcare provider, a one-day fast is recommended. However, preparations prior to and after the fast are equally important.

    a. One day prior to the planned fast, mentally and physically prepare yourself for the fast.

        i. Mentally: set the date and the time, e.g., from Thursday at 7 PM to Friday at 7 PM. Prepare yourself as to what you will do when you would normally eat during this time. Examples: Take a nap, take a short walk, read, do errands, clean, etc.

        ii. Physically: purchase and prepare foods prior to a fast and after the fast. Examples: a high-fiber diet with fresh fruit, vegetables, salad, vegetable soup, or water.

    b. During the fast, you may need to remind yourself not to eat, because it may be a big part of your life. Most importantly, pray; communicate with God. Remind yourself that you are loved. This is time for you and your body. So many times, you may take care of everyone else and their needs that you forget that *you* exist. You do exist. Keep reminding yourself that you are loved. This is communication that begins with the parent (conscious mind) and the child (unconscious mind/body). Note: take a bubble bath and wash every inch of your body and begin to rediscover the wonders of your body—skin, nails, arms, legs, toes, fingers, etc. You are wonderfully made. (Psalm 139:14)

LOVE SELF
SELF LOVE

Once you have communed with God and with self and realize that you are the temple of God, you want to feed yourself good things to keep your mind clear and focused. In addition, you want to keep this priceless gift (body) in good working order for the True Owner—God. You were bought with a price. (1 Corinthians 6:20)

c. After various fasting processes, some people go back to their old ways. **Turn this thing around!** Plan a nice light meal (e.g., salad without dressing—enjoy the crunchy foods and the true juices from the food). Allow your taste buds to send signals to your mind about the goodness of food—the wonderful gifts from God! Eat to live!

Through the fasting experience, you humble the once-dominating child who sees and wants everything. It is similar to a child who walks into a toy store and sees and wants every toy. Afterward, he begins to ask the parent with a sympathetic voice if he can take some toys home. Depending on the parent's circumstances and state of mind, the toys may be purchased. A fasting experience allows the person to experience the tremendous wants of the child (body). Every food or drink may smell and look good. Even the thoughts of favorite foods are desirable. The child's voice may be loud, demanding, and even distracting, to the point that the person wants to quit the fasting experience. Depending on the type and length of the fast, as time goes by, these strong thoughts and memories of food begin to dissipate. The voice of the child's wants becomes faint and then you are able to see and hear other members of the body—self-awareness. You are able to experience clarity by tapping into that spiritual power. Your child becomes humbled and has reached a point of listening. Balance—ground zero begins to set in.

Some items you may want to include in your salad:
romaine lettuce, nuts, salmon, avocado, raisins, boiled eggs, cauliflower, cucumbers, spinach, mushrooms, tuna, carrots, tomatoes, broccoli.

Some fruits you may want to eat:
Apples, cantaloupe, kiwi, mangoes, bananas, melons, grapes, apricots, peaches, strawberries, oranges, plums, blueberries, cherries, pineapples, honeydew melon.

Drink water according to your body's needs.

Appendix D

Support the Child

Every child needs support. They depend on the parent for everything. How will you support the child inside of you? The following are a few suggestions to support your child.

Pray to God
Communicate with God and tell Him your trials and tribulations. Praise Him. Sing songs and praises. Say your acknowledgment, truth and say it again statements throughout the day. Say a prayer—"pray without ceasing."[1]

Prayer Partner
Have you ever tried to turn on a lamp and noticed the plug was out of the socket? What did you do? Plug it in. Plug in to prayer with a partner, e.g., spouse, friend, mother, daughter, father, son, sister, brother, or cousins. Whenever two or more are gathered in His Name, He is there also.[2]

Light Friends
Have you ever tried to turn on a lamp and noticed that the bulb was out? What did you do? Change the bulb. You may need a change in support. Look around. Are your friends unconscious eaters? Sometimes, unconsciously they tempt you to eat things that are not good for your body. Be aware. Either make a stand with a parent's (conscious) voice to resist temptation of foods not good for your body or get new friends—light friends. Light friends are conscious of their lifestyle and may assist and support you in becoming a conscious eater. Sometimes they are role models both spiritually and physically.

Support Groups

There are two types of people who go to church: people looking for help and the others who have received help and are seeking to return the favor. Find a support group, Overeaters Anonymous, Taking Pounds Off Sensibly (TOPS), or others. You will find a treasure in support groups. This will be your Official Play dates!

Remember: Help someone once you have been helped!
Love your neighbors as yourself.[3]

Pictures/Reminders

Have you ever walked into a kindergarten classroom? You see lots of pictures and everything is labeled. The teacher helps the students to recite things over and over until they get it. For starters, cut out the acknowledgments and truths from the back of the book and put them on your refrigerator, walls, table, television, doors, mirror, etc. You are a child again. You will need pictures and reminders to reinforce your commitment to being a conscious eater and retrain your thought process and behavior.

Repetition/Meditation

Children must repeat words, rhymes, songs, multiplication, etc. until they get it. They must practice often and think about it daily until it becomes a part of them. The same practice works with spiritual food—the Word. The parent must train the child to repeat and meditate on the Word daily to resist temptations/lust of the flesh, including eating unconsciously. Become a child again by repeating scriptures and meditating on virtuous things so that you can resist the temptations of eating unconsciously. You will become more conscious and know how to respond to life's challenges.

Sharing

Sharing is something we teach our children at an early age. One, so they will not become selfish; two, so they will have a better appreciation of the things they have; and three to demonstrate their love toward others. Share with the homeless, a widow or widower, a child in need, or the poor. "In as much as ye have done it unto one of the least of these my brethren, ye have done it unto me."[4]

Play Time

Incorporating play time is essential to achieving a balance in one's life. Play time may consist of working out at the gym, playing volleyball, going bowling or skating, shooting pool, going for a walk, dancing, or doing something with the body that feels good to you. Anything that makes you feel like a kid again. Incorporate playtime into moments of your life. (Be careful!)

Scripture References
1. 1Thessalonians 5:17
2. Matthew 18:20
3. Matthew 22:39
4. Matthew 25:40

Appendix E

Affirmations

Are we there yet?

How do you know that you are becoming a conscious eater?

1. After your fast

During and after your fast, you may start to feel weak, even after eating your first meal. Now you are at ground zero. You are in a mode of "I need to eat to live." Do you remember Jacob and Esau in the Bible? Esau was starving so much that he sold his birthright for food.[1] Starvation is not recommended. This example is used to help you understand the purpose of food. Your body needs food for energy, to move, to think, to do, and to live!

You may have a better appreciation or understanding of why a hungry child cannot learn. Many children live in poverty, where fasting or starvation is prevalent. Children are expected to go to school to learn. However, if one cannot function without food, then it is senseless to ask the child to behave and grasp concepts at school. Thank God for the National School Breakfast and National School Lunch programs and the dedicated nutrition staff who serve children every day so they may learn and be educated.

Your affirmation is your body being aware of the struggle within, between the mind and body, ground zero—clarity is established, and the purpose of food is evident —"I need to eat food to live."

2. Look who is talking

In the beginning, you may find yourself talking out loud with the **acknowledgments, truths,** or **say it again statements.** This is okay. Communication between the conscious mind (parent) and the unconscious mind (child) is vital. This communication may occur several times.

Practice practice practice makes perfect. So practice until the child (unconscious mind) is trained up in the way it should go and not depart from it.[2] Eventually the child will get it and become conscious and the child will begin to do the right thing for the body (live, think, and eat consciously).

Have you ever found yourself talking to yourself? For instance, you forget to get milk while shopping at the grocery store. You say out loud, "Oh, I forgot to get the milk." It was the conscious mind saying to the unconscious mind, "Go get some milk!" Someone may observe you talking to yourself and smile. You may smile and say to them, "Oh, I was talking to myself. Don't worry, as long as I don't talk back, I am okay!" As reminders or affirmations, people recite reminders and affirmations all the time. So it's okay if the parent talks to their child—so long as the child does not talk back!

Your affirmation may be saying the **acknowledgment**, **truth** or **say it again** statements out loud on a regular basis until the actions desired become a natural habit.

3. You feel like a kid again and free

Eating becomes fun and exciting, and playing outdoors is exciting. You will find other life experiences that bring pleasure and put a smile on your face. You will realize that eating is only one part of the whole you. Your unconscious mind will have less energy to spend on just thinking about and eating food. You'll discover that there are too many other things to do in life than just eating. Sometimes you may become so overwhelmed with your purpose in life that you forget to eat. Then that faithful child/ baby gives you that cue of hunger and reminds you (parent) that it's time to eat—so you can eat to live and keep doing all the things that you enjoy. Suffer the little children for such is the kingdom of God.[3]

Your affirmation may be getting out of the comfort zone of mundane activities and preparing new recipes and/or going somewhere different to play and have fun.

4. New purpose in life

Hopefully your new purpose comes alive—to love God with all your heart, mind, soul, and strength and to love your neighbor[4] as yourself, whatever this means to you.

What is your talent? What is your purpose in life? At the end of this life, when people see you at your funeral for the last time, what memories will people have of you? Yes, they may have read that "she accepted Jesus at an early age," then what? What life did you live? What purpose or goal do you have in mind? Are you fulfilling that purpose? What do you want people to say about you or remember about you? What do you want your Creator to say about you? What will you do in a lifetime? Do you have charity? Will you continue to fight this spiritual and physical battle and put this body under subjection? Will you endure until the end? What will you overcome? Are you a good and faithful servant? When you ask yourself some of these questions, hopefully you will know your purpose in life.

Your affirmation is knowing your purpose in life and start making progress to live it as God directs you. Write it down and refer back to it regularly.

5. Feeling good

You now have a better concept of feeling good. That old man is crucified.[5] You have put off the old man and put on the new man.[6] "Therefore, if any man be in Christ, he is a new creature: old things are passed away; behold all things are become new."[7] "Cast away from you transgressions, whereby ye have transgressed; and make you a new heart and a new spirit: for why will ye die, O house of Israel? For I have no pleasure in the death of him that dieth, saith the Lord God: wherefore TURN YOURSELVES, and LIVE YE!"[8]

Conscious eating feels good. You know what foods to prepare for your body; you know how much to eat for your body; you know when enough is enough; and you know the meaning of being comfortably full. Now practice this over and over until it becomes a regular part of your life. This will make you feel better. You want to feel good.

Many people buy over-the-counter drugs and prescriptions for digestive disorders—because they *don't feel good*. Advertisements tell you to eat spicy and/or fried foods or overeat at a restaurant—"make yourself feel bad and this drug will make you feel better." Why do we go to an all-you-can-eat buffet and eat beyond our heart's and stomach's content? This is abusive to our bodies, this is physical abuse. Would you sit a child down and demand that he eats four plates of food—salad, two entrées, a dessert and two soft drinks? Why would you do this to *yourself?*

I beg you to turn it around. *Find out what foods your body is able to tolerate without gas, bloating, heartburn, diarrhea, constipation, and excessive fullness, and eat those foods!* You will feel good and your body and mind will thank you! Our bodies are so accustomed and addicted to feeling bad that feeling good may feel **abnormal,** and feeling bad and taking over-the-counter drugs to rid yourself of the pain is **normal.** We are so addicted to pain and agony that we tolerate it. This mentality is upside down like potter's clay – like the child that instruct the parent.[9]

You want to feel good. Your body enjoys feeling good. Once you know how to feel good, then things that make you feel bad—heartburn, coughing or choking after eating too much or too fast, chronic yeast infections, tooth decay, breathing hard with simple activities, constipation, gas, hemorrhoids, gout, tight clothes and shoes, headaches, bad breath, fatigue, sleep apnea, asthma, joint problems, depression, backaches, chronically tired, sleepy, etc., will feel strange. Your desire to feel good will override the feeling of feeling bad. Then you will know the meaning of "It feels Good to feel Good!"

The next time you go to an all-you-can-eat buffet, you will have a new concept in your conscious mind. "Eating at this restaurant will not make me feel good. I want to feel good! I know what makes me feel good!"

It is better to obey than to sacrifice.[10] A good child has happy parents; a disobedient child gives much grief to his parents. Have a sound mind and body and learn to eat consciously. Allow your mind and body to be happy and to feel good.

Your affirmation is knowing the bad feelings that your body experiences; being able to say "Enough is Enough!" and practicing conscious eating so that you may feel good.

6. Parent/child relationship is established

A parent of a young child always seeks to provide for that child, simply because the young child is unable to do for him or herself. For example, a parent of an infant may go to the mall. The parent will bring change of clothes, diapers, wipes, milk, and food. Or, a parent who takes a toddler on a day trip will bring a change of clothes, favorite toy, and snacks for the road. In each case, the child is innocent and humble and awaits guidance and support from the parent. Also, the parent is prepared for accidents, play time, and eating. Likewise with your body—your child awaits your guidance and support from the mind (parent). Forethought and planning should occur daily for the needs of the body, including eating. The parent (mind) that consciously plans will establish good and desirable eating habits for the child (body).

Your affirmation is becoming conscious of the body's needs, developing a track record, and planning meals for the day or week and having them available for the child who needs energy to continue playing.

7. Redirection of stress

During a period of stress, an unconscious eater may nibble on food throughout the day and not even **realize** how food and the amount that is used to calm a person's stressful situation or problem (similar to a chain smoker). When you have taken on a conscious lifestyle of eating, meditations, or physical activity, then you are better able to redirect your stress in a healthier way. Mediations may consist of visualization of secret moments in time, a favorite song hummed softly, deep breathing or a scripture or daily quote that gives a person hope and victory. Physical activity may consist of walking around the block during lunch, going to the park or gym, playing with children, doing yard work, dancing to a favorite tune, or doing chores around the house. Whatever the activity, whether it is meditations or physical activity, food is not the focal point. Food is only a source of energy to *live* and not to cope with stress.

Your affirmation is recognizing that foods are not used to relieve stress. You will find other ways to cope with your stress or life's challenges. Also, you will begin to accept life's challenges as lessons to yourself and examples for others.

8. Track Record

You have researched a track record that is meaningful to you and applied it to your daily living. Just as you would go to work and know what is expected of you on your job, you will know what is expected for your body—the child that has been given to you to take care of. Your track record consciously reminds you of the things that are needful for the body. Any new job may be challenging at first and then you become an expert on your job as time passes by. Likewise with your new track record, you will be challenged in the beginning, but eventually you will become an expert on taking care of this body. If you get off track, you will at least have a guide to lead you back to the track and live a life with a purpose.

9. Changed Attitude

A new attitude and confidence emerges when conscious eating is practiced. A sound mind and body become one, and the schism of that old man (mind wants to do one thing and the body does another) dissipates. Your attitude becomes one of self-love, such as following the airplane survival protocol. When the airplane is in danger, the passenger is instructed to first put on the oxygen mask, then assist the child or other passengers. In times past, you may have taken care of everyone else's needs, problems, and wants at the cost of you suffocating.

Now you have turned that thing around. With the new attitude, you now take care of yourself first, so that you can then begin to take care of others. Instead of absorbing traffic rage and hollering at a person who wants to cut you off in traffic, you in turn may smile, wave, blow a kiss, and even say a prayer for them. In past times, this may have set off an inner rage of eating unconsciously, but now the rage and stress is redirected, and self-love emerges to love God, the one who created you and your neighbor. A song or a thought of praise may be on your mind before, during, and after the situation.

Your affirmation is when you take care of yourself and your light begins to shine; you establish a new attitude; others maybe drawn to you and come to appreciate and respect your lifestyle with a purpose. You may even begin to be a role model for others – salt of the Earth.[11]

10. A spiritual transformation – growing a garden[12-23]

You are exercising spiritual muscles you did not know you had before. You are encountered with trials and tribulations and seek spiritual guidance versus food. You are overcoming the challenges of life. You have a desire to release the stress in new and different ways than in the past. Instead of eating to deal with challenges you are accepting the challenges and learning from life's lessons. Also, you are tucking those experiences away so that you can help some one else in this life journey. God's Word is steadily being revealed to you and your desire to read and meditate on God's Word becomes natural and apart of your life.

You start to laugh like a child because of this new found awareness and an acceptance of challenging experiences. The child is not in control anymore. Instead, the child is humbled like a sheep and follows directions versus giving direction. The CHILD obeys the voice of the PARENT. The BODY obeys the voice of the MIND. Harmony is established because the UNCONSCIOUS mind is now the CONSCIOUS mind – A RENEWED MIND.

Just as you would admire new clothing or hairstyle in the mirror, now you see and admire the spiritual body that is growing both physically and spiritually. You are beginning to form this new person that you like to see. The old man with the confusion, disorder, and dry bones is dead. Your house of chaos has been cleaned and it is in order. Your maturity has allowed you to put away childish things. The new thing, the new spirit and mind is being created and is alive inside of you with love, peace, joy, order, blessings, and light – God's kingdom is inside of you. You see your role and purpose in the BODY of Christ: to love Him with all your heart, soul, mind and strength and to love your neighbor as yourself. Now you see that you are created in God's image.

You begin to see that being close to God is a joy and delight. You want to testify of God's love toward you. You want to share the new thing inside of you. You are a seed that falls on good ground, a tree that bares good fruit to be shared with other members in the Body of Christ. You are a light to others and salt of the Earth. God's *will* shall be done in your Earthly body and it bares a grain for that Heavenly body. You now see that it is all about GOD and becoming a part of and building up the God family (creation/garden/kingdom). It's all about God!

Scripture References

1. Genesis 25:29-34
2. Proverbs 22:6
3. Mark 10:14
4. Mark 12:29-31
5. Romans 6:6 Colossians 3:3
6. Colossians 3:10
7. 2 Corinthians 5:17
8. Ezekiel 18:31-32
9. Isaiah 29:16

10. 1 Samuel 15:22; Mark 12:29-34
11. Matthew 5:13
12. Romans 6:6
13. 1 Corinthians 13:11
14. Romans 12:2
15. Isaiah 43:19; 2 Corinthians 5:17; Ezekiel 11:19-20
16. Galatians 5:22-24
17. Deuteronomy 28:1-14
18. Matthew 5:16
19. Luke 17:21
20. Colossians 3:10
21. Mark 12:29-31
22. Isaiah 58:13-14
23. Matthew 13: 3-9; 24-30; 37-38
24. Matthew 12:33
25. Matthew 5:13-16
26. Matthew 6:10
27. 1 Corinthians 15:35-49
23. Genesis 1:26-31; 2:1-3; Colossians 3:1-24

Appendix F

Don't Make Assumptions

Assumptions

In this book, many assumptions were made that the reader has Christian beliefs and/or American values. This book is a guide. You are encouraged to think of your own beliefs and values and put them into acknowledgments that are familiar to you. Also, write down visual examples of the acknowledgment. In addition, use your beliefs and values and put them into truths and statements. You are encouraged to speak them out loud, but if mentally is better for you, this is okay. Daily affirmations are important. Affirmations are essential to change and empower your current thought process.

Health Professionals

Your health professionals have specific training. They have a flashlight view of how you should overcome certain conditions, illnesses or disease, including being overweight. They make assumptions all the time: they *practice*, meaning some of it is guesswork. Why do you spend fifteen to thirty minutes, if that long, with a health provider who knows very little about you, your culture, values, and beliefs, the lifestyle that you live day in and day out? Then you expect a miracle to happen. Miracles do happen. However, oftentimes it is similar to a parent who has relinquished her responsibilities to the teacher and says, "Make my son or daughter a genius!" The teacher-student relationship is good because the teacher has the ability to positively impact a child's future, yet the teaching is limited (flashlight view). The parent raised the child from infancy and knows the values, beliefs, and education they want the child to have (overview). So, why does the parent relinquish this responsibility to the teacher? The parent is asleep (unconscious). Wake up! Wake up and take control by guiding, leading and training your child along with the teacher/health professional. This can be accomplished by empowering yourself to know more.

Avoid having the same expectations about your health, and say to the doctor, "Make me healthy or skinny." Before you arrive at your next clinic visit, write a list of questions and concerns to discuss with your healthcare provider. When you leave the office visit, ask yourself if all your questions were answered. Did the healthcare provider assess you appropriately? Were you empowered to go home and implement the necessary recommendations? Will you change your ways? It is not the healthcare provider who will cure you of your chronic disease, obesity or overweight, overeating. They cannot change you. It is *you*—the conscious mind. Be truthful in your assessment from your healthcare provider and be truthful to yourself and your commitment to being a healthy individual, including eating consciously.

Hopefully the healthcare provider will respond adequately to questions from a flashlight view. But it is up to the parent (conscious mind) with the new information to apply what's best for the child (body). Don't assume the doctor can read your mind or even ask you the right questions to assess your problem. Take control—the power is in your conscious mind.

Don't make assumptions about this book. It is only a flashlight view of a bigger picture. Hopefully this book draws you closer to your conscious mind and allows you to see the light that is in you.

"While ye have light, believe in the light, that ye may be the children of the light".[1]

"Ye are the salt of the earth: but if the salt has lost his savor, wherewith shall it be salted? It is thenceforth good for nothing, but to be cast out and to be trodden under foot of men. Ye are the light world ... Let your light so shine before men, that they may see your good works, and glorify your Father which is in heaven".[2]

Scripture References
1. John 12:36
2 Matthew 5:13-16

ACKNOWLEDGMENTS

ACKNOWLEDGMENTS

ACKNOWLEDGMENTS

ACKNOWLEDGMENTS

ACKNOWLEDGMENTS

TRUTH

Statement

TRUTH

Statement

TRUTH

Statement

TRUTH

Statement

Appendix G

Awareness of Self, Knowledge of Self, and Skills for Self

What are your struggles? (Awareness of Self –become aware of your struggle(s) and who you are as an individual including your strengths and weaknesses)

_____
_____
_____
_____
_____
_____
_____
_____
_____
_____
_____
_____

What is your purpose in life? (Knowledge of Self – define your purpose and diligently seek knowledge to fulfill that purpose)

_____
_____
_____
_____
_____
_____
_____
_____
_____

What is your **TRACK RECORD?** (Skills for Self – develop a track record that includes an eating or life plan tailored for you. Oftentimes, we have a mental note of what we should eat or do. However, writing down your track record will help you to stay on track! This book has some resources to assist the reader in establishing a track record. Establish a track record and practice these skills)

Appendix H

Can I talk to you?

A. Discussion Questions

1. Describe Illustration 1 on page 74.

2. How are your eating habits similar or different to illustration 1?

3. Describe Illustration 2 on page 75.

4. How are your eating habits similar or different to illustration 2?

5. Describe Illustration 3 on page 76.

6. Assess your lifestyle habits and compare it to both houses.

7. Assess your health and compare it to both houses.

8. Assess your spiritual life and compare it both houses.

9. Describe Diagram 1 on page 83.

10. Compare your health and spiritual habits to the map.

11. Describe Diagram 2 on page 87.

12. Describe Diagram 3 on page 87.

13. Where are you in your journey of conscious eating both physically and spiritually?

14. What areas in your life need improvement?

15. What does self governance mean to you?

16. What is a good steward?

17. What type of fruit do you bear?

18. What rooms in your house need cleaning?

19. What areas/rooms in your body/car need cleaning?

20. When your coworkers, friends, family or strangers think of you, do they think YOU are the salt of the earth, a good seed in the ground, or a tree that bears good fruit?

B. What do you see?

- Draw a picture of yourself

- Draw a picture of yourself eating unconsciously and describe your feelings

- Draw a picture of your self eating consciously and describe your feelings.

- Draw what you see around you related to unconscious and conscious eating.

C. How do you feel?

Describe how you feel when you eat specific foods? Does your body feel Good or Bad? Describe your feelings when you eat a specific food?

Food	Good	Bad	Feelings, i.e. mood, discomforts, etc.

Food	Good	Bad	Feelings, i.e. mood, discomforts, etc.

Appendix I

Did you get it?

Now tell me what I said?

Now it is your time to express yourself. Summarize any portion of the book and tell it to someone else. When you are able to express portions of this book that are meaningful to you and then share it with someone else both through your thoughts and actions, then you have ownership of the concept. Congratulations -You got it!

NOTES

NOTES

MEDITATION SCRIPTURES

MEDITATION SCRIPTURES

CONSCIOUS THOUGHTS AND ACTIONS

CONSCIOUS THOUGHTS AND ACTIONS

AFTERWORD

If you find yourself out of control physically, mentally or spiritually; or you have made excuses about life situations; or perhaps you have known you were out of control but felt helpless and could not do anything about it – then, this book will help you gain control. It will aid you in discovering the root cause of your problem. In it, you will find gentle, user-friendly support that will help you to get on the track to recovery and lead you to a wonderful fulfilled life that many only dream about. -- Viola T. Miller

OTHER SUGGESTED READINGS

Miller, Viola T. (2005) *Check Yourself.* Trafford: Victoria, BC Canada.

Taylor, Earl W. (2009) *Overcoming Yourself: A Journey Towards Self Improvement and Oneness.* iUniverse: Bloomington, Indiana.

Other References

Harris-Davis E, Stallman I. Nutrition in Public Health. In Edelstein S, ed. Addressing Overweight in Children: A Public Health Perspective. Sudbury, MA: Jones and Bartlett Publishing; 2005.

Harris-Davis E, Haughton B. A Model for Multicultural Nutrition Counseling Competencies for Registered Dietitians. *J Am Diet Assoc.* 2000;100:1178-1185.

Sue D, Bernier J, Durran A, Feinberg L, Pedersen P, Smith E, Vasquez-Nuttall E. Position Paper: Cross Cultural Counseling Competencies. *Counsel Psychol.* 1982; 10:45-52.

Sue D, Arrendo P, McDavis R. Multicultural Counseling Competencies and Standards: A Call to the Profession. *J Multicul Counsel Dev.* 1992; 20:64-88.

ABOUT MY PARENTS

My parents, Elbert and Dorothy Harris were my first teachers in life. My dad taught me at an early age about conscious eating. Although I did not know it at the time, he taught me about physical and spiritual eating. Physically, I remember him visiting the health food stores or markets and bringing home delightful fruits and nuts and other items I would try for the first time. In addition, I remember my dad chewing his food forever before he swallowed, and actually rejecting food when he was full. (Also, he exercised on a regular basis). Spiritually, I remember my dad quoting one of his favorite scriptures on a regular basis, "Wisdom is the principal thing, therefore get wisdom: and with all thy getting Get understanding" (Proverbs 4:7). My mom made weekly Sabbaths special for our family with family worship on Friday nights and hosting frequent gatherings after church with family and friends. In addition, she gave advice all the time, whether you wanted to hear it or not, and always stood up for what was right. Both of my parents have a sincere love for family and friends, and they give from their hearts. They have been a blessing in more ways than one to me and others. However, one thing I appreciate about them the most is that they talked to me regularly and they were loving, honest, and forthright in guiding me during my youth. Because of this, they wanted me to make wise decisions and avoid unnecessary pitfalls, pains, and agony in life. Each generation should be stronger than the last. My parents provided a strong foundation for me and my siblings. I hope in my lifetime, I will be able to lay one good stone in God's foundation. Also, I hope the messages in this book are loving, honest, and forthright in guiding my sons and others to become stronger than *me*.

Thanks, Dad and Mom.

P.S. The apple does not fall too far from the tree.

ABOUT THE AUTHOR

Edna Ellen Elizabeth Harris-Davis is a Registered Dietitian with Master of Science and Master of Public Health degrees. She has enjoyed several career opportunities throughout the years: extension agent, nutrition manager, research dietitian, grants manager, television producer, nutrition coordinator, health educator, and author, along with several volunteer opportunities. More importantly, she enjoys celebrating the Sabbath days, writing and spending time with family and friends.

She developed a love for the Sabbath and writing at an early age. At one time, she had 15 pen pals all over the world through a church magazine for teenagers. Today, she has one pen pal/sister of 26 years.

Nutrition and diet were always fascinating to Mrs. Davis because of her own diet practices through her church teachings. Later, she pursued a BS degree in nutrition/dietetics. Although there is a science to nutrition, she realized after 17 years of practice that there was something missing when you look at the overweight and obesity problem in the United States today. While the scientific side of nutrition and eating is good, the spiritual/conscious side is rarely talked about. Maybe because it is spiritual— the unseen thing—that few people want to address it.

Mrs. Davis set out to write about nutrition, health, and consciousness, however, it became more evident to include spiritual aspects as it relates to this topic. Physical food is just as important as Spiritual food – God's Word. The Bible is an instructional manual and it teaches you how to care for your mind and body – the true inward man or woman. God's Words are Spiritual and they provide the peace, harmony and serenity that some individuals are seeking when it comes to overcoming the struggles with food or any other challenges in life.

Mrs. Davis hopes that readers will embrace conscious eating: physical food for the body and spiritual food for the soul. "Beloved, I wish above all things that thou mayest prosper and be in health, even as thy soul prospereth." 3 John1:2

Mrs. Davis has been married for 12 years and has two sons.

_ LOVE CHILD _